Caring in Nursing Practice

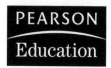

We work with leading authors to develop the
strongest educational materials in nursing,
bringing cutting-edge thinking and best
learning practice to a global market.

Under a range of well-known imprints, including
Pearson Education, we craft high-quality print and
electronic publications which help readers to understand
and apply their content, whether studying or at work.

To find out more about the complete range of our
publishing, please visit us on the World Wide Web at:
www.pearsoned.co.uk

Jacqui Baughan
Ann Smith

Caring in Nursing Practice

PEARSON
Education

Harlow, England · London · New York · Boston · San Francisco · Toronto
Sydney · Tokyo · Singapore · Hong Kong · Seoul · Taipei · New Delhi
Cape Town · Madrid · Mexico City · Amsterdam · Munich · Paris · Milan

Pearson Education Limited
Edinburgh Gate
Harlow
Essex CM20 2JE
England

and Associated Companies throughout the world

Visit us on the World Wide Web at:
www.pearsoned.co.uk

First published 2008

ISBN: 978-0-273-71460-6

British Library Cataloguing-in-Publication Data
A catalogue record for this book is available from the British Library

Library of Congress Cataloging-in-Publication Data
Baughan, Jacqui.
    Caring in nursing practice / Jacqui Baughan, Ann Smith.
         p. ; cm.
    Includes bibliographical references and index.
    ISBN 978-0-273-71460-6 (pbk.)
  1.   Nurse and patient.   2.   Empathy.   I.   Smith, Ann.   II.   Title.
    [DNLM: 1.   Nursing Care--psychology--Case Reports.   2.   Empathy--Case Reports. 3. Nurse's Role--Case Reports.   4.   Nurse-Patient Relations--Case Reports.   5.   Nurses-- psychology--Case Reports.   WY 87 B346c 2008]
    RT86.3.B38 2008
    610.7306'99--dc22

                                                                    2008035584

10 9 8 7 6 5 4 3 2 1
12 11 10 09 08

Typeset in 9pt Interstate light by 30
Printed in Great Britain by Henry Ling Ltd., at the Dorset Press, Dorchester, Dorset.

For all the people who contributed their stories and reflections: service users, carers, students and qualified staff. In particular, this book is dedicated to the memory of Janine and June.

We have changed the names of people in the stories to maintain confidentiality but you will recognise yourselves. We are also grateful to all those who helped us to bring this book into being, including colleagues at Northumbria University, and Kate at Pearson for her enthusiasm, guidance and support.

Contents

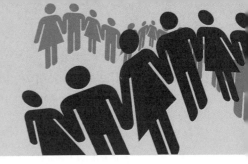

Preface

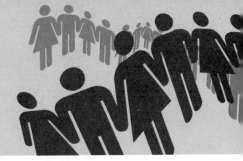

In the pressurised and rapidly changing world of health care it is increasingly important for nurses to maintain and extend their capacity to be caring. Although the notion of caring is seen to be at the very heart of nursing, much has been written about the difficulties in defining exactly what this means. Attempts at doing so by using difficult and abstract rhetoric may complicate rather than enlighten. We have drawn on our long experience in practice and nurse education to write a book which is grounded in the reality of everyday practice. We did not expect to arrive at an all-embracing definition but would like readers to see the book as a means for embarking on a journey of exploration to uncover indicators of the many dimensions of caring. We saw an urgent need to enter into this dialogue as nurses may be in danger of perhaps dismissing or undervaluing the complexity and importance of their caring attitudes, knowledge and skills. In this book there is evidence that those being 'cared for' see a caring nurse as making a valuable difference to their care experience.

We believe that an effective way of exploring the notion of caring is to use stories from practice as a focus for our reflection. We were very fortunate and privileged that student nurses, qualified staff, service users and carers gave us their rich and engaging stories as a basis for our exploration. Without these, the book could not have been written and we owe the contributors our deep appreciation and gratitude. We have changed the names of people in the stories to ensure confidentiality but they will recognise themselves.

The stories from students and qualified nurses helped us to identify significant caring moments in practice that occurred not only in busy traumatic periods but also in everyday situations. Other stories from people about their lived experiences of illness or disability, in being cared for or providing care, helped us to identify important indicators of caring partnerships. They helped us to recognise the significance of professionals being only one small part of a continuum of care.

The first five chapters of the book are concerned with the nature of caring relationships and provide indicators of attitudes, knowledge and nursing interventions which assist or which can be detrimental to care partnerships and therefore of effective care provision. Throughout the book there are 'thinking clouds' and other reflective exercises which aim to help readers relate to their own experiences. The focus of the book changes slightly in Chapters 6 and 7 where there is more emphasis on what individual nurses might do to recognise and increase their capacity for caring. In the final part of the book we review what we have learned from the caring indicators, and these are summarised in Chapter 8 within the BOND framework as a means of reflecting on the nature of caring. In the final chapter the importance of continuing the journey of identifying the dimensions of caring is emphasised so that in the future the value of caring knowledge and practice will not be lost. We found the stories we used both awe-inspiring and humbling. We hope you will find the same and that you will continue to see your own stories and those of your colleagues and patients/clients as a rich resource for your future personal and professional development.

In summary, this book is about the art of caring within nursing practice. It is primarily aimed as a guide for student nurses who are at the beginning of their professional life. However, it will also be useful for mentors and other qualified health care professionals who support students or for those wondering whether to embark on a career in nursing. Support workers, who are such an integral part of health and social care teams, may also find it helpful.

Jacqui Baughan and Ann Smith
June 2008

Acknowledgements

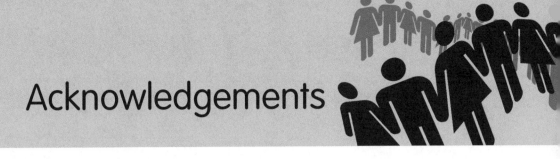

We are grateful to the following for permission to reproduce copyright material:

p. 9, excerpt from Eliot, T S (1963) 'Little Gidding' in *Four Quartets*, reprinted by permission of Houghton Mifflin Harcourt Publishing Company, copyright © 1942 by Eliot, T S and renewed 1970 by Esme Valerie Eliot,; Excerpt from 'Little Gidding' in *The Wasteland and Other Poems* by Eliot, T S, published in 2002 reprinted by permission of Faber and Faber Ltd; p. 32, from Redwood, S (2004), Case study 3: Careers in nursing research. In Freshwater, D and Bishop, V (eds), *Nursing Research In Context. Appreciation and Professional Development*, pp. 130-131, reprinted with permission of Palgrave Macmillan; p.38, excerpt from Smith, S (1972) 'Not Waving But Drowning' in *Collected Poems of Stevie Smith*, reprinted with permission of New Directions Publishing Corp, copyright © 1972 by Stevie Smith; pp. 124-125, adapted from McKergow, M and Clarke J (2005) *Positive Approaches to Change: Applications of solutions focus an appreciative enquiry at work*, with permission of Solution Books.

We would like to thank the reviewers for their helpful and constructive comments that have helped shape the book:

Sue Bowers, Staffordshire University
Andrew Evered, Swansea University
Sheila Mealing, London South Bank University
Sharon Urwin, Kingston University

Chapter 1
Creating a caring discourse

LEARNING OBJECTIVES

By the end of this chapter you should have an understanding of:

1. What caring might mean to nurses and service users
2. How stories can be used as a focus for reflection
3. How our reflections can help us to create a caring discourse which will enable us to begin to unravel the complexity of caring
4. How key indicators, such as being available, using informal social exchange and 'connecting' with service users, can point us to ways in which we can improve our nursing practice

Introduction

In this chapter, we will introduce storytelling as a means of discovering what caring is all about . We will show how theories can be beneficial and exciting in helping us to shed light on our experience and that of service users and their families. Our discussions will lead to new meanings and understandings - in other words help us to create a caring discourse and add to the evidence base for your practice. From those discussions we will begin to identify caring indicators, to which we will add more in later chapters. We can use these to strengthen the way we care in practice.

We will discuss ways in which you, as a student nurse, can make a valuable contribution to the creation of a caring environment. We look closely at the notion of compassion in caring, the complexity of caring and the potency of nursing presence. We will consider ways in which we are able to 'connect' with patients and the long-lasting impact of emotional feelings. We will discuss how we can use and share stories as an important basis for reflection and to help us to identify key indicators of caring practice.

Caring at the heart of nursing

Do you see caring as at the very heart of what you do as a student nurse? It was probably the most important reason that brought you into the nursing profession in the first place. However, you may well think that your acts of caring are under pressure in a health care system which has increasing challenges and pressures. You are not alone in this. The Nursing and Midwifery Council (NMC) has recognised the need to respond to public and professional concerns by including care, compassion and communication amongst its Essential Skills Clusters (part of the Standards of Proficiency) which must be integrated into every pre-registration nursing programme (NMC, 2007). Approaches such as this help us to understand the expectations of our patients and clients, and to gain the skills and qualities needed to provide quality care. We still feel, however, that a deeper understanding about the nature of caring through an exploration of its many different aspects and presentations will assist us even further in achieving this, and this is the purpose of this book.

We have called this chapter 'creating a caring discourse' which is our way of summarising what we see as an exploration through storytelling of what caring really means to us as nurses and to our patients/clients and their families. We all tell each other stories about what we felt about various situations we have come across at work. In these stories we express our emotions, thoughts, knowledge, judgements, ideas and values. In other words, like us, after a hard day's work, you probably have the need to go through your highs and lows and let off steam with someone you trust. It is these stories that make up a shared nursing discourse. The term discourse is used to describe the way particular groups of people talk about their shared experiences. For example think of the ways adolescents talk to each other, which is very different from the way they might talk to their parents! In our work, there is also patient/client discourse and medical discourse. In this book we are using stories from people who have been involved in providing or receiving care to help create a caring discourse. The stories will be used as triggers for our discussion and we will draw on academic and other literature to gain more insights and to broaden and deepen our understanding.

We are drawing on experience gained over a number of years during which we have been studying the subject of caring by collecting critical incidents from patients, students and registered nurses (written and verbal accounts of significant events in their professional careers). We have found that many aspects of caring are unrecognised by nurses themselves but accepted as expectations of the role, rather than as something special. These caring moments have occurred in busy and traumatic periods and also during 'everyday' situations. We have also found evidence of the importance of the ability to express caring behaviour, illustrated by the guilt and frustration nurses feel if opportunities to engage in meaningful relationships with patients and relatives are thwarted. Have you felt like this too?

How students can make a valuable contribution to the creation of a caring environment

In our rush to get through our everyday work, we may forget that it is in very simple ways that caring can be expressed. Have you thought about the contribution students can play? Let us consider a message sent by a relative to staff about the care her grandmother had received from Jo, a student nurse in her first placement.

Case Study 1.1

'From a relative's point of view with absolutely no experience of hospitals I didn't have a clue where to go for advice, who to ask for information or what jobs each person I came into contact with did. Jo was wonderful because she was approachable. I used to visit Gran twice a day and whenever Jo was around she would have a chat with Gran. The chat might just be, "Hello Alice. How are you today?" But she never walked by without saying something which meant that Gran and I got to know her. Although I knew that Jo was a student and as such had no authority I realised very quickly if I asked her something she would find out the answer and let me know as soon as possible. I felt that some of the more senior members of staff were too busy to deal with what they considered to be "trivial" questions. Jo treated my Gran the way she would treat her own Gran and nothing was too much trouble for her.'

Have you had a similar experience as a student nurse? If you have been singled out for a particular mention in a 'thank you' card or in verbal communication, have you considered why? Reflecting back will increase your ability to pinpoint what you did that was particularly valuable, so that you can use opportunities to repeat this in the future. You can increase your caring skills even more if you use academic knowledge in this reflection. This is what evidence-based practice is all about. Our discussion below will help us to demonstrate this by reflecting in more depth and exploring Jo's contribution to the quality of Alice's experience of care.

Using theory to understand practice

The caring behaviour of the student was recognised and appreciated by both Alice and her granddaughter. Jo, inexperienced and in her first placement, conveyed warmth and interest ensuring that both perceived they were important to her and that what they asked was of consequence. In short the student was sending out a powerful message – that she cared – and she did so by using her natural warm, informal communication skills which are an important part of social exchange. The contribution student nurses make to creating a caring environment is not a new discovery but can be found in studies of nursing practice, e.g. Morrison (1994: 91) noted that students were 'singled out for their attentive care and devotion' and thought their constant availability was particularly appreciated by the patients.

Student nurses have excellent opportunities in all branches of nursing to provide holistic care and make real efforts to listen to and attend to individual needs. It is sad that more experienced and qualified health care professionals may be so preoccupied with competing demands on their time and energy that they may not be so easily available for providing the kind of contact that service users and their carers seek. Although students are in a position where they can develop close relationships with patients and relatives, a difficulty is that because of their lack of nursing experience, they may not always know how to respond effectively in complex situations (Dowling, 2006).

Have you found yourself in this situation? It may be reassuring to know that other students have found this too and that, in spite of the situations in which you now feel out of your depth, you will gain confidence and become much more skilled over time. In the meantime however, don't be afraid to tell your mentor or supervisor how you are feeling because he/she is there to help and guide you. Indeed, they will probably share with you their similar experiences as a student.

Sadly, it could be that when opportunities for assessing and attending to individual needs arise, all grades of nursing staff fail to take them. For example there have been debates within the profession that some highly qualified nurses (and also some students) may be missing out on opportunities to engage in caring activities which may occur whilst providing intimate or fundamental care. It has been argued that core nursing tasks have been devalued (highlighted in the 'Too posh to wash' debate (Wright, 2004) and nurses have distanced themselves from these, focusing instead on high technological or management roles. Although organisational and economic pressures and skill mix decisions may have resulted in fewer opportunities for 'hands-on' care, it is reassuring that experienced nurses such as Freshwater and Biley (2005: 14) question the assumption that nurses think themselves too superior to undertake such tasks, saying that '... our own experiences as nurses on a variety of busy wards were quite the opposite. We enjoyed being able to escape to the patient; those hours spent behind the curtains managing 'basic care' provided the ideal opportunity to engage in what was for us central to nursing: the therapeutic relationship'.

The centrality of caring to nursing has been there since the profession was established but it seems to be the one thing that might be so easily lost, diluted or undervalued as other priorities take precedence.

Time to think back

+ What do you think?
+ Do you think you make the best of the opportunities when you help patient/clients with fundamental care needs?
+ Have you found that some patients felt able to talk about their fears and concerns when you have been providing what may be described as 'everyday' care?

Students and health care support workers are important resources. Valuable communication exchanges between patients and relatives and qualified staff may be affected by restricted opportunities, professional status and demanding role responsibilities. As we have seen in Jo's story, patients and relatives may be anxious not to burden more senior staff with what may seem to them to be 'less important' matters so instead they may approach the student or support worker. The relationship Jo had with Alice and her granddaughter was helpful and supportive, benefiting from the opportunities they had to become familiar and comfortable with each other through the informal social exchanges that took place during their encounters. Ersser (1997) has described the value of 'natural' emotional exchanges. Students like you and Jo, often do see the worth of these forms of communication when they begin their careers and perceive these 'natural' emotional exchanges as an essential component of being able to 'care'. Being able to help people is, for most, the main reason for coming into nursing in the first place and becoming 'distant' is what many say they are most fearful of (Smith, 2003).

An added problem is that the very nature of caring may not be understood, as we shall go on to examine in the rest of this book. Caring may be taken for granted as something that comes naturally, particularly for women, but its complexity (for example the emotional as well as the physical skills required), may be underestimated (Smith and Gray, 2001). Compassion is an integral part of this and if we are to give effective patient-centred care of the kind we would want the closest members of our families to receive; we need to look for ways in which this is demonstrated.

Looking more closely at the compassion in caring

Consider the following story to gain insight into how a patient might experience compassion from a student nurse. Harry, a 50-year-old businessman, described his hospital experience:

Case Study 1.2

'I was in a medical ward after a heart attack. I've always felt in control of situations and hated being ill. I think I coped with this by making myself the life and soul of the ward. I'd chivvy up the other men and we'd have a laugh about what was happening to us like going to X-ray wearing backless nighties! When my family and friends came in we'd talk about football and what was going on 'outside'. I talked to my wife about the tests and treatment and she spoke to the doctors and nurses. When she was there I did my best to make everything seem normal. One night I woke up and couldn't get back to sleep again. Rashida, a student nurse, noticed I was awake and asked me if I wanted a cup of tea. When she brought it, she must have noticed something was wrong because she asked me how I felt and for some reason I started to cry. I couldn't stop and I felt so stupid.

I said to her, "Everyone thinks I'm coping but I'm not!" She just sat and held my hand. I told her that I didn't want my wife to know that I wasn't really a strong person. It's hard to know how long I wept but it seemed as if she sat with me for a long time and not only then but several nights after she would come and sit with me for a while when it was quiet in the ward and we'd talk about how I was overcoming some of the fears I had of dying and leaving my family. I'm very appreciative of all the care I had – you couldn't fault the medical care I was given. I had full explanations of everything but when I look back I still remember that time in the middle of night and how much that student nurse's presence meant to me.'

To think about

+ Think about what we can learn from Harry's story about the nature of presence as part of compassion.
+ Think about a situation in your practice. Reflect on how your presence has helped someone who was frightened or anxious.

You might want record this within your ongoing assessment record /practice portfolio. Remember to use pseudonyms to protect patient confidentiality.

Harry's story helps us to understand the importance of holistic care and shows that the emotional features of care are as important as the rest of the knowledge and skills required to care. It illustrates how important it is to be 'available' to give supportive care (not just technical care), and to have a 'caring presence'. This is what can be described as showing compassion. It also demonstrates the opportunities for care which nurses working at night can have. Kirby and Slevin (1992: 73) cite Marcel who, writing in 1949, spoke of the nature of real presence:

'The person who is at my disposal is the one who is capable of being with me with the whole of himself when I am in need; while the one who is not at my disposal seeks merely to offer me a temporary loan raised on his resource. For the one, I am a presence, for the other, I am an object.'

Harry did not feel he was treated as an object. We can infer this because Harry was able to tell the student nurse of his fears. Perhaps this was easier for him to do than to tell his wife because he would have been less worried about upsetting her. Rashida was able to show that she cared only because she spent time with Harry, held his hand and waited for him to talk but she also followed this up by being available on subsequent occasions. These may only have been for a few minutes but would have made Harry feel that his feelings continued to be seen as significant and he would have felt more comfortable with his disclosures.

Roach (2002: 28) has helped to deepen our understanding of the nature of human caring and describes caring as a natural capacity of human beings. She emphasises that it is 'not an exceptional human quality, nor the response of an exceptional few. ... It is the most common, authentic criterion of humanness.' This is perhaps is why students, even with little professional experience, can be so good at it. Roach (2002: 71) reaches the conclusion that people use occupational roles to express their natural, and self-fulfilling, human capacity to care. She describes this as the core value since, 'it inspires, directs and sustains nursing's identity and the identity of all persons who choose professions of care.'

Rashida entered nursing with a really useful resource – the capacity to show compassion. The important issue to consider is how we use our 'natural' human capacity to care within our practice and also what may stand in the way of how we can develop and extend it. It may not be as straightforward as we may initially believe.

The complexity of providing care

Many nurses aim at becoming highly skilled in technical tasks and being able to engage in sophisticated interventions, whilst for others it is the ability to engage in more fundamental care which gives them greater career satisfaction. Allan (2001) points to the disagreements various authors have had on the type of caring which patients and nurses themselves value and the degree to which different forms of caring are thought to be effective. As a consequence of these disagreements, she points to the continuing debate between those who see the emotional component of caring as its most defining feature and those for whom the practical aspects are more important. It is interesting that Tarlier (2004) insists that this kind of debate about the relative importance of different caring skills has stopped productive discussion and, rather than helping, it has been at the expense of understanding the complex nature of nursing.

To think about

+ Think about your care of a particular person.
+ What caring skills were you using?
+ Do you think some were more important than others?

You will find your answer will be influenced by a variety of factors depending on the urgency of the situation, the most pressing needs of the patient/client or their families, and so on. Reflecting back on the situation, were there any other caring skills you wish you had used?

Did you find it difficult to say that one skill was more important than another? If you had asked your patient, would you have got the same answer? It is therefore also a question of who is making a judgement about what was important about the care. Patients or relatives may have a very different perception of the situation. Even in life-threatening situations where rapid physical interventions are vital, communication skills between team members and with the patient are also essential. For us, the debate about the relative importance of each skill has limitations but uncovering the often hidden, caring dimensions within care delivery will help us more in our understanding of what effective, holistic caring is all about. In other words, we are searching for what puts the caring into care.

As a student nurse, you are likely to have been aware of the high emotional feelings that caring for someone can bring and have wondered whether you responded in the best way. Have you ever been left feeling uncomfortable, challenged and emotionally, as well as physically, drained? On the other hand, have there been times when you found your nursing experience very exciting and interesting and have gone home knowing that you have done a good job, perhaps that lives have been saved or improved and clients and relatives appear grateful. At these times you probably feel that all is right with your world! It is a wonderful feeling when you enjoy nursing and appreciate caring for others! Perhaps these highs and lows contribute to the excitement of nursing and make it one of the least boring jobs.

As we have discussed, to unravel the complexities of what we mean by caring practice, there is a need for a degree of reflectivity or time to mull things over. Over the past few decades much emphasis has been put on reflective practice within the context of holistic, individualised care often described as the ideology of nursing practice (ideas of what nursing is or should be). This kind of care brings with it many challenges. Each individual is unique and has distinctive physical, psychological, social and spiritual needs. For example, try to imagine a situation in which a young man called Jimmy Jones is admitted to an accident and emergency department (A+E) with a paracetamol overdose and a diagnosis of alcohol abuse. A holistic caring approach will consist not only of managing the serious life-threatening event but also of finding ways of providing ongoing help in such a manner that Jimmy feels recognised and valued as a human being in every interaction with health care professionals. This will need the integrated, thoughtful, patient and non-judgemental approach of an interdisciplinary team.

Nurses contribute to the care within an effective team. Faugier (2005: 19) suggests that 'when the unified force of experience, intellect and passion come together within a skill like nursing, it transcends the ordinary as much as a Michelin chef or a Ryan Giggs goal'. So, whilst a magnificent goal in football or the production of an excellent meal is most likely to be the combination of experience, knowledge and practice, the use of intelligence and the application of skill, it also depends on motivation and enthusiasm. Good nursing care often calls for a complex mixture of ingredients. In Jimmy's case, excellent holistic care requires the application of a range of knowledge (for example, amongst other things, the science of the human body, the psychology of dependency, legal aspects and ethical frameworks) and practice skills (assessments and interventions likely to overcome a life-threatening event, risk assessment and a range of longer-term interventions). But these alone do not make care complete. Knowledge and skills need an essence of caring applied in an artistic way such as through the use of self and self-awareness or creative responses to meet individual needs. We think that this sort of care is what people mean when they say that good nursing combines both art and science. This sort of care can create a feeling in the recipient that someone has gone that 'extra mile for them'. It is what changes a good nurse into an exceptional nurse.

Dunlop (1986) describes caring as a public form of private love and this may well come close to the rewarding aspects which many nurses entering the profession say they hope to experience. It would seem however that special experiences of care, may not, in Faugier's terms, be 'sensational goals' which may be dramatic and unexpected but instead be an integral part of an everyday experience in which patients needs are really met.

The potency of nursing presence

We have already seen how the presence of both student nurses, Jo and Rashida, demonstrated caring communication and compassion and was a powerful or potent influence. There are times, however, which unfortunately we all come across, in the hustle and bustle of everyday practice, in which some caring aspects are missing. Consider the following story given to us by Julie, a relative, and think about why she was so upset. What did one nurse do which made all the difference?

Case Study 1.3

'My mother was seriously ill and although we felt that the nursing staff were polite, they gave us minimal attention and information and we thought that they were not really wanting to listen to us. I guess that they might have believed that they were giving good enough care but to be honest, it wasn't really good enough for us as they were not really available and seemed to be avoiding us. One evening when we were feeling particularly despondent, a bank nurse came into the room. She stood for a moment and then asked us how we were and how Mum was. It was the first time we felt that someone cared and really wanted to help. This gave us the opportunity to say what we were worried about – which was how Mum's pain was being managed. The outcome was that within hours a Macmillan nurse came and Mum became pain free for the first time for days. Thank God for that nurse!'

From Julie's story it seems that in general the nurses' world of care was far removed from what Julie and her mother needed. The nurses focused on what they perceived as the pressing activities and may even have thought that they were giving good care or they were so immersed in the ward routine they weren't thinking about individual patient needs. It is interesting that in telling her story, Julie saw as particularly significant the action of the bank nurse who 'stood for a moment'. This nurse gave the impression of availability. She was summing up the situation and was in a state of readiness to listen. That simple act made all the difference in the implementation of effective care and it is this kind of action that we need to consider and extend. These examples are in line with Barker's (2003: 9) suggestion that an important way of considering care is with an emphasis on 'caution, attention to detail and sensitivity that is necessary when handling something precious'. He draws parallels with the work of an archaeologist who adopts a 'care-ful' strategy for unearthing and revealing a possible find, including sensitivity and attention to detail.

Actions may be unthinking if they are part of routinised procedures. The actor and playwright Alan Bennett (2005: 12) wrote about the impact on him of what he describes as 'the casual cruelties that routine inflicts' when visiting his mother who had just been admitted to a psychiatric unit. 'She had on admission been bathed, her hair washed and left uncombed and uncurled, so that now it stood round her head in a mad halo, this straightaway drafting her into the realms of the demented. Yet the change was so dramatic, the obliteration of her usual self so utter and complete, that to restore her to even to an appearance of normality now seemed beyond hope. She was mad because she looked mad.'

These stories point to the danger of routines which dehumanise or of a chaotic rush of activity and preoccupation, both of which lead to loss of individuality and a danger that patients and their relatives or friends feel they are overlooked or ignored. A nursing presence is likely to provide a potent caring indicator in that the nurse acknowledges the intrinsic worth of each individual.

Time to think back

So far we have uncovered indicators about what Alice, Harry and Julie saw as important aspects of caring and also what they saw as unhelpful. We can use these positive indicators as pointers or signposts to guide us on our journey in creating a caring discourse. For example, we saw that just being there and being emotionally available can significantly improve patients' and relatives' experience of care. You will uncover more indicators through reflections on more stories as you progress through the book and we will use these to gain a fuller picture of the components or dimensions of caring. Since reflection is such an important part of this process, we will spend a little time looking closely at how we can use stories for this purpose.

Using stories to create a caring discourse

Stories create vivid images which remain with us and help us to learn. We know from our own and others' experiences, that we repeatedly recall certain specific moments that have had an impact on us. You will have recounted these moments as stories, or anecdotes, to others because they are meaningful to you. In simplistic terms, we reflect back on our experiences. As Schon (1983) notes, this is 'reflection on action' and in your nursing programme you will be directed to using reflective models as a means of helping you to learn most from particular situations which have occurred in practice. Stories help us to look again at a situation and find new meanings and understandings. Our nursing students have found a quotation from a poem by T S Eliot (1963: 222) very useful in summarising the impact of new discovery within a familiar situation:

> *'We shall not cease from exploration*
> *And the end of all our exploring*
> *Will be to arrive where we started*
> *And know the place for the first time.'*

We can use stories as the means for furthering our journey of exploration into caring and because stories are an important part of everyday life – they form a vital way of communicating with and relating to each other. We hear stories every day in our workplace and they can have an important impact on our individual practice. What we learn from them may guide and influence us, in our ways of working and influence our beliefs, values and expectations. However, if we use these stories without reflecting on them, we may build up nursing myths, some of which may be helpful and some less so, e.g. the myth that nurses should not become emotionally involved.

By using stories as a focus for our reflection we can critically explore myths, beliefs and values and so increase our knowledge of caring by building up a caring discourse. It is important that we also include stories from those being 'cared for' as we will then be more knowledgeable about their perceptions of the caring process and so be in a better position to learn from and transform nursing care. We have to be sure that the resulting discourse is one in which questioning occurs and assumptions are challenged and one way of achieving this is through shared, critical discussion.

Phillips and Benner (1994: vii) reiterate the importance of sharing caring narratives. 'We believe it is essential to recover the vision of what is possible in actual practices today.' These nursing academics think that through the knowledge gained by sharing actual experiences we will able to have a greater impact on future policies and decisions about how care is provided. This emphasises the importance of sharing and learning from experiences – so something we may undertake on a daily basis can be turned into a truly learning exercise.

The best of circumstances offer conditions for learning, and reflections can be about happy experiences and moments that have made us feel successful and competent. However, there may also have been times when we are anxious, shocked, sad, angry, guilt ridden and fearful and when we have been greatly puzzled by our own and others' responses, leaving us with unanswered questions. As a student, you are likely to encounter a number of these moments in nursing and you may tend to share these experiences with individuals who are important to you, perhaps colleagues who understand you and with whom you feel safe. On the other hand, there are times when you may have difficulty in discussing them for a variety of reasons. You may think that others may judge your thoughts, questions, feelings or actions since in sharing something personal we put ourselves at risk of judgement. Stories, therefore, have another important feature which needs to be taken into consideration.

The way we tell and reflect on our stories depends on who is listening to us. As Mishler (1991) says, any story is socially reconstructed and reflects the content and the expected audiences. A case in point: your reflections as part of your educational course or in clinical supervision are likely to take on a different form from 'storytelling' occurring with a colleague in an informal setting. Whatever form it takes, however, we can learn from storytelling. Stories are linked with our self-image, or ways in which we see ourselves. They help us consider the role we are 'playing' in a particular location.

Smith (2003) suggests that storytelling, as part of the reflective process, can help nurses test out possibilities for future behaviours and help refine and/or integrate ideas about various concepts. She came to this conclusion by using the research method of narrative analysis, which led her to focus on trying to discover the moral of the stories nurses told, as students and as graduates, in other words, why they told particular stories in the first place. This approach helps to identify significant phrases such as the one Julie used ('*she stood for a moment ...*'), which are particularly important to the individual telling the story but can easily be missed. Julie, whose mother needed pain relief, told the story because she wanted to convey the way in which the bank nurse gave time to the family and picked up their distress. The impact of changes in Alan Bennett's mother's appearance highlighted by the phrase '*She was mad because she looked mad*', emphasises the impact unthinking 'routines' can make, in this case in reinforcing a stereotype. This approach points to the benefits to be gained from writing down stories and looking at them in more depth.

We have found that using written stories from students and qualified nurses has helped us over a number of years to understand practice better (Smith and Russell, 1991; Smith and Russell, 1993). We used them in workshops where participants were able to compare their hopes and fears with those of others and also they provided an opportunity for us all to gain increasing awareness of what can inform and influence future nursing practice. We are increasingly aware of the importance of also using stories from service users.

To think about

Write a brief story based on an incident from your practice which made an emotional impact on you:

+ Just write as if you were telling the story to a trusted friend.
+ Underline any phrases which you see as particularly significant.
+ Think about why the story was important to you.
+ Consider what you have learned and how this will affect your future practice.

You might like to keep this as part of your reflective learning diary or ongoing assessment record.

Sharing stories with others

Sharing stories can be very helpful, as was illustrated by Vicky, a newly qualified nurse, who brought the next incident to one of our reflective workshops. She wrote about an important and frequently questioned aspect, that of 'having emotions' when caring for patients. As you will see, Vicky ended her written account by wondering whether it is acceptable for a nurse to cry. She indicated that she had asked herself this question as a student but even years after it still remained an issue for her. Sharing it helped her understand the complexity of caring and why the question had remained with her for so many years. We think it is one you too may be asking yourself!

Case Study 1.4

'I was a newly qualified nurse and the consultant, the house officer and I approached an elderly gentleman, called Henry, who had been frequently admitted to the ward with heart failure. Henry seemed a warm-hearted man and had made an impression on me. The consultant said, "I am sorry we have come to the end of the line; we have talked about this before, your heart is not strong enough to recover this time." I was shocked as I had not realised his heart failure was so 'end stage' and that he was so poorly. The two doctors left and I looked at Henry who started crying. What should I do?

I sat on the bed next to him and began to sob too. Henry gave me a hug. He told me that he believed in God and that he wasn't frightened of dying. I felt he was comforting me, but surely it should be the other way around? Eventually I left him. The senior nurse took me into the day room. He said it proved that I was human and that nurses have feelings. I did feel a little better, but felt that crying may not have been the best way of handling this situation. After all a nurse can't cry; can she?'

This story illustrates the uniqueness of the encounters between patients and professionals. In this instance, nurse and patient shared an intense, close and significant moment. It seems that Vicky's main focus is on finding a correct way of responding in the situation. Nurses should not cry! Nurses can cry! We think that the story illustrates the type of questions that nurses ask themselves but one to which they often fall short of finding a simple and satisfactory answer. It is difficult to articulate what is expected of a nurse, a 'caring professional'. Could it be that there is no simplistic correct answer to this and other similar questions?

Using reflection to increase our understanding

By reflecting, or looking again at the story, we can see that this newly qualified staff nurse, in trying to make sense of the situation, is unlikely to find an 'ultimate truth'. In order words there will not be one straightforward answer. This does not mean reflection is not helpful but that it helps us to come to terms with the nature of knowledge that is often incomplete and uncertain. Work by Carl Rogers (1978) might help us understand this. He suggested that there is no such thing as a static truth but instead truth is about a series of changing approximations – we make judgements based on our varied experiences and perhaps limited knowledge.

Different perceptions and views of the same events are illustrated by the clinical psychologist Pamela Stephenson, who is the wife of comedian Billy Connolly. Pamela writes about her husband's disturbed, abusive and dreadfully poor childhood in Glasgow and notes how he survived and triumphed over this. In the introductory remarks in her book (Stephenson, 2001: 1), she recalls her emotional reaction relating to the tremendous effect these circumstances would have had on him, and notes Billy's retort to her emotional response was, 'Well, I didn't come down the Clyde on a water biscuit'. Perhaps this story demonstrates that whatever events occur, traumatic or otherwise, there are different perceptions and understandings to be made about their impact and the influence. She pointedly says: 'for every one life, there are a million observed realities, including several of the subject's', so talking this over may have made them both think again and see things in a new light.

In summary, to explore the story of Vicky's response to Henry it is helpful to reflect by using a wide variety of perspectives and in doing so, try to gain a 'best fit' understanding of the situation at hand. 'Factual' answers (answers that can be claimed to be completely scientific, objective, accurate and applicable/transferable to all circumstances) may at times be difficult to find. Although clear evidence and rational explanations have a vital role in care situations and interventions, many aspects of practice cannot be easily explained by applying a theory which covers all aspects of unpredictable human situations. We can therefore, as an alternative, look for literature, perspectives or theories, in order to help illuminate, or shed light on, what Schon (1987) describes as the unpredictable and 'swampy world of everyday practice'.

Nursing in the dark

An early but influential qualitative study by Melia (1987) revealed some very interesting ideas about what it is to be a nurse. Her study with student nurses concluded that they learned to 'get the work done', 'learn the rules', 'nurse in the dark' and 'be professional'. Using her work can lead us to reflect on the similarities in the situation the newly qualified staff nurse found herself in, still wondering whether or not it was really all right to cry in front of a patient and speculating about what her work really should involve, trying to learn and/or remember the rules about being a professional.

This seems to be what is happening to Vicky. Whilst the incident is occurring she begins to ask herself what she should do next when Henry starts to cry. Sharing this incident with colleagues in a reflective session, helped her to see that she was almost unthinkingly using good communication skills when she sat next to Henry to try to comfort, or reassure him. Someone suggested that she started to sob due to a 'heavy personal attachment' she had for Henry and another questioned whether this was a good thing to have. Others disagreed and asserted that, by crying openly in front of Henry, she showed him that she cared about him and this displayed a characteristic of a caring nurse.

Most of her colleagues at the workshop thought that showing emotions as part of a caring approach is beneficial and an aspect of a therapeutic approach to care (and in written reflections later were able to draw on references in the literature to back this up: e.g. Peplau, 1952; Leininger, 1978; Barber, 1991; Ersser, 1997; Dowling, 2006).

However, as you can see in the incident, at the time Vicky felt uneasy, as if she sensed these were not, as she saw them, the 'rules' of everyday professional practice. Despite being given a form of reassurance from a more senior nurse, she continued to feel that she might have handled her emotions in this situation in a different way. In the discussion group, her colleagues inferred from her final comment, '*After all a nurse can't cry; can she?*', that Vicky was not clear about the 'rules' in this situation. From their discussions they concluded that showing emotion is an important aspect of care but were aware that this could be overwhelming at times. Talking over the incident with colleagues and gaining perspectives from literature helped them become more aware of how common such emotions are. Freshwater (1999: 29) confirms the benefits of this approach, suggesting that reflection provides an important opportunity 'for caring individuals to explore and confront their own caring beliefs and how these beliefs are executed in practice'.

We have seen the importance of reflection in increasing our understanding, so if you look for ways in which theory can help explain and analyse practice, it will not only help to ensure you meet the academic requirements of your course but more importantly it will become an integral part of your ongoing development as a nurse so that the quality of the care you provide is increased. It can also help you gain in confidence. Smith (2003) found that reflection helps students and qualified nurses to become more confident in their ability to react to changing circumstances, including the ways in which they demonstrate caring. We all have a tendency to become static and unadventurous by clinging to that which we feel safe and comfortable with and so may be reluctant to reflect. Such an approach can have dire consequences for us all since without learning from the past or the present, we cannot explain what nursing is all about and we may be prone to ritualistic and unthinking care so that good care is compromised and the 'freedom' to progress is lost. We may, for example, not be aware of the importance and impact of the way in which we 'connect' with patients.

Time to think back

+ Have you ever felt out of your depth and overwhelmed in terms of your emotional response to situations?
+ Did you cover up your feelings or did you talk to someone else?
+ You wouldn't be alone in feeling like this. One of the skills that you will learn is how to handle close relationships within professional boundaries. You may find that talking to your mentor/supervisor or someone you can trust, such as fellow student, will help. Others find that using a reflective diary helps to look again at the situation and see things in a new light, such as understanding why you felt so upset.

Connecting with patients using emotional labour

Just like you, many nurses have meaningful moments with their patients during which time a very close connection is made which may have been quite emotional. Nursing theorists, such as Parse (1992), explain the importance of patient and nurse co-creating the unique human experience of illness, within a relationship of 'connectedness'. Smith (1992) captures the essence of this when she quotes a patient who praises the nurses who held her hand 'both literally and metaphorically'. However, the closeness of some of our relationships with patients and their families can seem quite challenging.

Nurses have to learn to cope not only with the task in hand but also with the emotions that sometimes threaten to overwhelm them as practitioners. A number of authors, such as James (1989) and Smith (1992) use the phrase 'the emotional labour of nursing'. The demands of emotional work can be equally as hard as physical and technical labour, but not so readily recognised and valued although it has a key role in the creation of a caring environment (Smith and Gray, 2001).

Smith (1992) drew on the work of the sociologist Hoschild, describing emotional labour as requiring 'surface and deep acting' which nurses learn to use when there is a gap between what they do and what they feel. Have you ever tried to cover up your feelings in practice? You may have made a determined effort to appear calm when a patient is angry or seems hostile or you may have overcome feelings when encountering distasteful smells? What you are doing then is surface acting in which you consciously change a facial expression to show a particular emotion that you want others to perceive. In deep acting we change the feelings inside us by, for example, conjuring up images, so that we show the feelings we want the other person to see. For example, we might imagine that it was our relative or friend we were caring for so that we then display more caring attitudes. Good actors are adept at intentionally manipulating thoughts, feelings and behaviour so the purpose of emotional labour and 'acting' is to produce an outward appearance which helps in the connectedness of the relationship.

Connecting with patients and being yourself

In something of a contrast to labouring with our emotions and 'acting' in response to these, another early study by Jourard (1971), is helpful to our deliberations. He asserted that nurses need to learn to 'be themselves' with patients. He said that genuineness and congruence (what is being portrayed by our actions corresponds to that which we feel internally), warmth and positive regard are important in demonstrating that we care for others. Jourard believes that nurses should find ways of expressing themselves and their emotional concerns – rather than hiding or denying them – and sums this up in his phrase 'The Transparent Self'.

Self-awareness and the therapeutic use of self are identified as key requirements for effective interactions and connectedness. To see how this relates to practice, if you return to the incident with Henry who was given bad news, we think Vicky was showing her 'transparent self', her emotional concerns were not hidden or denied, but rather 'congruent' with her behaviour. She cared about him and she showed this, but was very concerned that this was not the right way to behave, perhaps wondering if it would have been better (that is, more therapeutic) for Henry, if she had laboured emotionally and in her terms 'acted in a more professional' manner. Probably the best answer would have come from asking Henry what his perspective of the situation was! However, we believe that this nurse was able to give Henry something very precious by caring for him in this transparent and congruent manner.

The nature of closeness or intimacy within the therapeutic nursing relationship and the ways in which this is managed will be an important aspect of our discussion in the following chapters. Another aspect which we will also return to later, concerns another interesting question that Vicky asks when she wonders if it is appropriate for Henry to offer some sort of comfort to her – the 'professional'. It seems that she is expected to be the provider rather than the receiver for this relationship to be therapeutic.

Have you experienced something like this in your practice when you have been frustrated because you wanted to be able to give a 'perfect' response in an emotional situation? What we have learned is that we will rarely be satisfied with what response we give but the emotions engendered may stay with us for a long time.

The long-lasting impact of emotional feelings

Even if you have been in nursing a relatively short time, you can still probably remember the emotions you felt in your first days in practice? Some of these will probably stay with you for a long time. Sean, who gave us the following story, says he remembers an incident vividly, even though it occurred many years ago. He is now a university lecturer and says he relates this story to students who struggle with guilt feelings and unanswered questions when they cry in front of relatives. It helps us to explore further the impact of emotional feelings concerning patients to whom we particularly connect.

Case Study 1.5

'My first post after qualifying was on a trauma intensive care unit. I was on duty one afternoon when John was admitted with severe head injuries following a road traffic accident. It soon became apparent that the injuries John had sustained were so serious he would not survive. His parents were informed of this and were obviously very upset at the news. I was allocated to look after John and his parents; they spent a lot of time at John's bedside and we talked about his treatment. His mother also asked questions about my life and during the discussion we determined that I was only four days older than John. This somehow seemed to help his mother. The following day I was again allocated to care for John. His mother brought some photographs of him and showed them to me and talked of John – what he was like, his job and his friends. Over the next few days of caring for John I felt I got to know him very well through his mother.

A few days later I came on to the ward to discover that John had died. His parents came in and his mother put her arms around me and cried openly. The emotion was so intense that I also cried. We exchanged few words, as they weren't really necessary. That night when I got home I lay on my bed and cried. I was really upset that John had died. Even though we had never spoken, the discussions I had with his mother made me feel that we had known each other all of our lives. My mother came into my bedroom and asked what was wrong and when I told her she said she could not understand how I could be so upset over someone I had never really known. I did know him, even if he did not know me!'

Sean says that he believes the incident taught him that it is important to 'be you' and not try to hide emotions. Because he behaved in a congruent manner in that his feelings and behaviour matched and he did not try to 'act the professional part' (whatever that may actually be) he showed he cared about John and his parents. Sean thinks that this helped the parents, especially John's mother, to grieve for their son. As for himself, Sean says:

I often wonder what John's voice sounded like. I really felt I knew him, although I never even heard him speak. The fact that he was so close to me in age also had something to do with why his mother got close to me and I got close to John. It was as if I did know him.'

This raises an important question. Why is it that with some patients we feel as if 'a button is pressed within us' and we feel more linked into their lives, deaths, problems and issues? Fosbinder (1994) describes this as 'clicking' – an immediate rapport between patient and nurse – which facilitates the process of 'getting to know you' but can also lead to the uncovering of some deep emotions within us. Perhaps some situations may be more significant and even problematic for us because the situations somehow remind us of someone who has died or from whom we are now parted or we worry about losing someone close to us. It may also be that we become more aware of our own mortality. Reflecting back on such situations can lead us to a deeper understanding and acceptance of ourselves and others.

Summary

All these incidents, stories and scenarios are rich, potential learning experiences and are the beginning of our journey into the development of what we hope will be a useful caring discourse. This has already led us to raise many questions and explore some of the key issues such as:

+ The importance of understanding and developing the skills of caring for nurses and their impact on service users.
+ How stories can act as a focus for reflective discussion and for showing how theoretical perspectives can provide us with an evidence base for practice.
+ The identification of aspects which are sometimes overlooked or underestimated, for example the importance of 'being there', of a caring presence. These indicators can point us to ways in which we can improve our nursing practice.

Looking forward

We will build up a collection of such indicators at the end of each chapter. At the end of the book all these caring indicators will be used as indicative criteria for a framework of caring. This framework will help us to know more about the dimensions of a caring approach, integrating compassion, empathy, concern and kindness within a context of skilled, informed evidence-based nursing practice. In the next chapter we will continue our journey by considering what else goes on within a caring relationship by exploring what we receive from, as well as what we give to, caring relationships.

Activity

Look at the caring indicators. Use them as you think will be most beneficial, for example:

+ Apply them to your practice and note when you have done this.
+ Consider how your actions and reflections can help you towards attaining some of the outcomes and proficiencies set out in your nursing programme.

Caring indicators

1. A caring presence – being available for patient and family
2. Participating in informal social exchange
3. Listening and using non-verbal cues
4. Connecting to patients and significant others
5. Recognising significant rapport (e.g. 'clicking') and its effects on our responses
6. Willingness to enter into a reflective discourse in order to learn
7. Noticing effects of interactions
8. Responding and attending to detail in a 'care-ful' way
9. Labouring emotionally when required
10. Displaying authenticity
11. Not allowing routines or business to 'blot out' individual care

References

Allan, H (2001) A 'good enough' nurse: supporting patients in a fertility clinic. *Nursing Inquiry* **8**, 51–60.

Barber, P (1991) Caring: the nature of the therapeutic relationship. In Jolley, M and Perry, A (eds) *Nursing: A knowledge base for practice.* London: Edward Arnold.

Barker, P (2003) Person centred care: the need for diversity. In Barker, P (ed) *Psychiatric and Mental Health Nursing: The craft of caring.* London: Arnold.

Bennett, A (2005) *Untold Stories.* London: Faber & Faber.

Dowling, M (2006) The sociology of intimacy in nurse-patient relationship. *Nursing Standard* **20**, 48–54.

Dunlop, M (1986) Is a science of caring possible? *Journal of Advanced Nursing* **11**, 661–670.

Eliot, T S (1963) *Collected Poems 1909–1962.* London: Faber & Faber.

Ersser, S (1997) *Nursing as a Therapeutic Activity: An ethnography.* Aldershot: Avebury.

Faugier, J (2005) Be proud of your skills. *Nursing Standard* **19**, 18–19.

Fosbinder, D (1994) Patient perceptions of nursing care: emerging theory of interpersonal competence. *Journal of Advanced Nursing* **20**, 1085–1093.

Freshwater, D (1999) Communicating with self through caring. The student nurses' experience of reflective practice. *International Journal for Human Caring* **3**, 28–33.

Freshwater, D and Biley, F (2005) Heart of the matter. *Nursing Standard* **19**, 14–15.

Kirby, C and Slevin, O (1992) A new curriculum for care. In Slevin, O and Buchenham, N (eds) *Project 2000: The teachers speak.* Edinburgh: Campion Press.

James, N (1989) Emotional labour: skill and work in the social regulation of feelings. *Sociological Review* **37**, 15–42.

Jourard, S (1971) *The Transparent Self.* New York: Van Nostrand Reinhold.

Leininger, M (1978) *Transcultural Caring: Concepts, theories and practices.* New York: Wiley.

Melia, K (1987) *Learning and Working: The occupational socialisation of nurses*. London: Tavistock.

Mishler, E (1991) 'Once upon a time …' *Journal of Narrative and Life History* **2/3**, 101-108

Morrison, P (1994) *Understanding Patients*. London: Baillière Tindall.

NMC (Nursing and Midwifery Council) (2007) *Essential Skills Clusters (ESCs) for Pre-registration Nursing Programmes*. Nursing and Midwifery Council Circular 07/2007.

Parse, R (1992) Human becoming: Parse's theory of nursing. *Nursing Science Quarterly* **5**, 35-42.

Peplau, H E (1952) *Interpersonal Relations in Nursing*. New York: Putnam.

Phillips, S and Benner, P (1994) *Crisis of Care*. Georgetown: Georgetown University Press.

Roach, M S (2002) *Caring, the Human Mode of Being* (2nd edn). Ottawa, Ontario: CHA Press.

Rogers, C (1978) *On Becoming a Person: A therapist's view of psychotherapy*. London: Constable.

Schon, D (1983) *The Reflective Practitioner*. London: Temple Smith.

Schon, D (1987) *Educating the Reflective Practitioner*. San Francisco: Josey-Bass.

Smith, A (2003) Learning about reflection. PhD thesis, Northumbria University, Newcastle upon Tyne.

Smith, A and Russell, J (1991) Using critical learning incidents in nurse education. *Nurse Education Today* **11**, 284-291.

Smith, A and Russell, J (1993) Critical incident technique. In Reed, J and Proctor, S (eds) *Nurse Education: A reflective approach*. London: Edward Arnold.

Smith, P (1992) *The Emotional Labour of Nursing*. London: Macmillan.

Smith, P and Gray, B (2001) Reassessing the concept of emotional labour in student nurse education; the role of link lecturers and mentors in a time of change. *Nurse Education Today* **21**, 230-237.

Stephenson, P (2001) *Billy*. London: HarperCollins.

Tarlier, D (2004) Beyond caring: the moral and ethical bases of responsive nurse-patient relationships. *Nursing Philosophy* **5**, 230-241.

Wright, S (2004) The value of values. *Nursing Standard* **19**, 15-16.

Chapter 2

Caring as a two-way process of giving and receiving

LEARNING OBJECTIVES

By the end of this chapter you should have an understanding of:

1. The benefits of rewarding partnerships in nursing care
2. What we gain from, as well as what we give to, those relationships, particularly from 'small' often unrecognised actions
3. The need to accept emotional gifts from patient/clients and appreciate the mutual benefits to be gained
4. The importance of satisfying relationships for informal carers

Introduction

In this chapter we consider the satisfaction to be gained from caring for others. Early images portrayed nurses as self-sacrificing 'angels' administering to the sick for no personal gain, but changes in nursing itself and the climate of professionalism and diverse career opportunities have done much to dispel that myth. However, understandably there is still a focus on what nurses give to service users in the kind of care they provide and less so on what they gain themselves from their relationships and care opportunities. The purpose of this chapter is therefore to explore the nature of mutuality (what we share) and reciprocity (what we give and receive) in our caring relationships as we work towards true partnerships with service users and their carers. It will help us to understand the care relationship better and what we achieve in rewarding or 'connected' relationships. However, as more care is being undertaken by family and friends in the community, we will also consider the relevance of this for them too. In this chapter, we will also return to a consideration of how we might use theory to help us explain what is going on in our working life.

Images of nurses

Nurses have been represented in many different ways. In the past they have been portrayed as 'ministering angels' illustrated in the image of Florence Nightingale as the 'Lady with the Lamp' providing comfort and help to wounded soldiers in the Crimea. This image was one of selfless-ness and uncomplaining service to patients and of subservience to the medical model of care. Other media images such as the 'dragon matron' and the 'sexy female nurse' also portrayed nursing in a particular light. These images influenced public perceptions of what nursing is like for a long period and probably still have some impact even today in spite of some more recent media attempts to overcome the stereotyping and portray a more skilled and professional image. Since the 1960s with the development of nursing knowledge and increasing moves towards levels of autonomy, independent practice and clear accountability, a strong growth in professionalism has emerged. It is important that nurses continue to be recognised as highly trained professionals, so that they are able to use their influence on the way care is provided and that they are financially rewarded in terms of salaries and opportunities for career development. However, the image of nurses as care-givers, although obviously true, may perhaps lead us to forget how much we ourselves gain from the recipients of the care we provide.

Perhaps you recognise this in your own experience in which your interactions with a patient or his or her family helped to make you feel good. For example, someone may have given you a special 'thank you' or even a word of encouragement when you were having a bad day. We think it will be useful if you continue to think about this as we move on in our exploration of caring because we see nursing care as a series of partnerships – in which we give but also receive. When we feel we are doing a good job and others recognise it, we get a boost to our self-confidence and gain the satisfaction of knowing that we are helping others. Perhaps though, there are days when things do not go so well. Can you think of times when you have been despondent and felt like a 'spare part'? This often happens to students when they begin their nursing programme when they see everyone else looking as if they know what they are doing. It is a common experience and may even occur later on. An exciting aspect of nursing is that you will be learning new things throughout your career. It may be reassuring to know that as your experience grows so too will your ability to adjust to and learn from new challenges.

Moving towards a rewarding partnership

Consider the following story told to us by Marjorie, a community nurse. Think about how she was able to turn a 'spare part' experience into a positive one, beneficial for both Sukwinder (the patient) and Marjorie herself.

Case Study 2.1

'Sukwinder had recently returned home from hospital following treatment for metastatic breast cancer. As her community nurse I visited her regularly, monitoring her symptom control, liaising with her general practitioner (GP), arranging for the installation of equipment and helping her to apply for state benefits. However, she appeared to be an organised, self-reliant individual. I began to feel that once the practical issues had been sorted out she did not really need me. I knew she had a strong informal support network as well as close links with the Macmillan nurse, the hospice and the hospital. Perhaps she considered me to be yet another cog in the wheel of the health service that she had to endure because it is the system. I felt increasingly uncertain about the value of these visits. Could it even be that my visits were detrimental to her well-being as I was a reminder of her illness and a disruption to her everyday life? Should I withdraw temporarily?

But, despite my misgivings I continued to visit. One day when I arrived, she was resting on the settee and complaining that her legs were swollen and heavy. Without really thinking about what I was doing, I knelt down and put my hands on her feet. They felt so cold. I instinctively started to rub her feet gently in order to warm them a little. I asked her if she had ever had a foot massage. She said, "No, not really but I like having my feet played with!" So I just rubbed and stroked her feet. At intervals she talked a little.

After twenty minutes or so when I had finished Sukwinder asked me if I would have time to do it the next time I came. I felt good about myself. I felt that I had eventually been able to do something to make her feel better.'

Time to think back

+ Have you ever found yourself in a similar situation or feeling irritated or frustrated because you never seem to be able to help some people enough?
+ Do you agree that Marjorie believed that it was important that whatever care she gave was seen as beneficial and valuable by Sukwinder? It was therefore a process not just of giving but also of receiving something in return, an acknowledgment that what she did was helpful and therefore provided positive feedback which made her feel good.
+ Can you apply this to the situation you thought about when you felt awkward or out of place?

You will be aware that not everyone makes us feel valued. Some people seem to make 'demands' on our time or are even hostile towards us. They may be doing so in response to their situation and we have to ensure that because we do not find it easy to care for them, or that they value us less, that we do not ignore them, avoid them or treat them unprofessionally. We will consider these difficult kinds of situations further in Chapters 3 and 6 but for the moment we will stay with the importance of feeling valued.

Achieving a connected relationship

In the story, Marjorie, the community nurse, was able to use an opportunity which presented itself almost instinctively. If she had given up and withdrawn initially, this would not have happened. Sukwinder gave her the opportunity to care both then and in the future. According to Roach (2002: 68), the connectedness of a relationship does bring with it certain responsibilities on both sides: 'Whenever we are in a relationship with another person, we establish bonds and these bonds, grounded in trust, entail duties and responsibilities – an ethic of relational responsibility.' What Roach is emphasising here is the importance of acknowledging that there are expectations on both sides of any relationship. In applying this to nursing, it is useful to consider what we expect from service users. These may be emotional gifts such as recognition of our capabilities, our skills and our qualities or perhaps it is in the way others respond positively to our suggestions or advice – all the 'feel good' factors gained from having been a help to someone else. We may also gain other gifts such as learning opportunities and even reassurance.

Marjorie's story also demonstrates other important aspects of relationship building. It shows if nurses concentrate only on negative features, such as the things they may feel unable to do or situations in which they perceive their ability to contribute is very limited, there is a danger of ignoring positive aspects. It shows that by relaxing and having an open and friendly approach, nurses may find new opportunities which they might miss if they are preoccupied with only doing or saying 'the right thing'. Perhaps in our drive to be seen as highly skilled practitioners, we forget about the value that basic human warmth and presence can bring. Barker and Davidson (1998: 351) stress the importance and benefits of this for mental health nursing:

> 'What little evidence exists suggests that when people become psychiatric patients, they would rather receive care than some sophisticated therapy; they require validation of their experience rather than processing for change; they desire an encounter at a fundamentally human level, rather than a carefully negotiated ... consumer–provider contract.'

Vivien Lindow (1996: 186) (who is a service user herself) reinforces this by writing about the difficulties people with mental health problems have communicating with professionals:

> 'One of the most persistent complaints about service users is "They never listen". But diagnosis and the effects of psycho analysis get in the way of listening. The medically inclined listen to the words of service users in order to diagnose: "Is she psychotic?" This robs our words of their meaning. The analytically inclined listen to demonstrate their skill in gaining insights. This again robs our words of their meaning. If we disagree with our clever analyst (or even therapist or counsellor) it demonstrates denial, projection, transference or one of the other 'mechanisms' that stop what we are communicating to be heard.'

We have to be careful that we do not resort to using professional jargon as a way of explaining and justifying our interventions. We also need to be aware of what is called the impact of meta-communication which demonstrates the complexity of communication and why it can so easily lead to problems. Using the example above we can illustrate this: Lindlow is thinking about what the professional is thinking about her thinking. She suggests that is problematic because they are using their own various frameworks as explanations rather than listening enough to her. You might like to read more about the complexity of communication since this is an area which causes most problems for service users in all areas of health and social care. It seems then that we have to be aware that establishing partnerships, which are built on trust and honest exchange, can be difficult with service users since many other aspects (although we may find them helpful), such as professional knowledge, expertise and an unequal power relationship, may cloud perceptions and even get in the way of clear and effective communication.

To think about

Think carefully about Vivien's story and what we can learn from it for our practice:

+ Think about what you have learned about what can get in the way of communicating with service users.
+ Think about your own area of nursing. You may be caring for adults, children and young people, or for people with learning disabilities. How is Vivien's experience applicable to your area of work? Do we sometimes jump to the wrong conclusions?

You might like to keep this information as part of your reflective learning diary or portfolio.

Using theory to help us explore the nature of patient–nurse relationships

We can expand our discussion about how we might achieve and maintain effective partnerships further by considering a study which was undertaken over a decade ago but from which we can still learn a great deal. This may help us to recognise and respond to those relationships which may cause problems.

Theory helps us to think about aspects which we might not otherwise consider. Morse (1991) undertook a research study of a variety of care situations from which she was able to describe two main types of patient–nurse relationships (mutual or unilateral). The first type she called mutual relationships which differ in terms of involvement and intensity and depend on a number of factors such as the length of time they occur, common needs and desires, and personality factors. These relationships are partnerships and mutually beneficial. There is a general agreement in terms of what is expected of each other and the kind of behaviour which may occur. However, the unilateral, or one-sided nurse–patient relationship, is characterised by asynchrony (people are out of step with each other) and this kind of relationship is likely to break down for a variety of factors. Perhaps this is because the nurse is unable or unwilling to see the patient as a person or if professional power is misused or its influence unrecognised. This can also occur because the patient does not understand or accept his or her condition, hospitalisation or treatment. Another reason for asynchrony is if a person has either a physical or a psychiatric illness which makes communication very difficult. The challenges of both recognising and overcoming such barriers are an essential aspect of the skill of caring if we are to achieve and maintain effective partnerships with service users.

Morse went on to describe various strategies used by both nurses and patients to increase or decrease the level of the developing mutual relationships. In her study, nurses used activities which showed an overt demonstration of commitment (giving time, anticipating needs, getting to know the family and being the patient's advocate) to increase involvement. On their part, the patients, first of all assessed whether the nurse was 'good' in terms of displaying empathy and kindness, had a confident and gentle touch and was dependable (technical competency is assumed) and they then also used strategies by being what they saw as a 'good patient', being friendly and joking or trying to be 'no trouble'.

Morse found that if the nurse wanted to maintain control (thereby achieving a relationship based on inequality or asynchrony), they tended to depersonalise the patient, avoid eye contact, maintain an air of busyness and not be forthcoming with information, keeping patient and relatives 'in the dark'. On the other hand, some patients also used powerful tactics in trying to keep control by preventing the nurse from 'knowing' him or her, such as avoiding conversations which were of a personal nature, talking only of symptoms and treatment.

Morse's study is still pertinent today in emphasising that the nurse–patient interaction is an involved process in which both participants are involved in 'giving' and 'receiving' and also that this is not a static process but ever changing. As in the Sukwinder story, some patients do not seem as if they want or need help initially but change as the relationship develops. It was 'commitment' which made Marjorie look for ways in which she felt she could help Sukwinder. Morse (1991: 467) also considered whether 'commitment' might be a more important and appropriate term to use than 'caring' in the nurse–patient relationship and preferred this as an alternative description, 'In the emotional sense, caring has notations of 'fondness' or 'love' neither of which may be present (or desirable) in a professional relationship'. However, perhaps rather than an alternative description, we would argue that commitment is yet another dimension of the caring process.

To think about

+ Think of a relationship with a patient/client in which you felt connectedness or mutual understanding. What were the factors which helped you to achieve this?
+ Think of a relationship with a patient/client which you felt was one-sided (there was asynchrony). What attempts were made or could have been made to overcome any negative consequences of this?
+ See if you can find parallels in your reflections with the Marjorie and Sukwinder story and/or with Morse's research study.

You might like to keep this information as part of your reflective learning diary or portfolio.

Recognising the contributions of service users to a connected relationship

Memorable interactions may illustrate how service users may help nurses to look at things in a new light and influence their relationships. Thomson (2005: 71) wrote about one such an event:

'I joined a team of nurses talking after the unexpected death of an alcoholic, homeless patient. They described how they had discovered a strong sense of fun in him when he taught some of them to dance. Their appreciation in him had increased his confidence, which in turn deepened their relationship with him – a magic moment.'

Through caring for others we gain many things. For example, Roach (2002) uses work by Mayeroff (1971: 30) to support this, suggesting that caring for others brings immense benefits to ourselves which we may not always recognise. 'By using powers like trust, understanding, courage, responsibility, devotion and honesty, I grow also; and am able to bring such powers into play because my interest is focused on the other.' Benner's (1984) important study of expert nurses also found that nurses benefited from what they did. They saw care as a two-way process and identified with their patients as active participants not as passive observers.

This may involve an ability to respond in a sensitive way on the nurse's part. Look at the following incident described by Jamie, a student nurse, and think about how the community nurse responded to a patient's comment:

Case Study 2.2

'While out on my community placement with my mentor, I visited a man in his early sixties. Jim was an alcoholic and was practically bedridden, due to lying in bed all day and having a very bad diet. He smoked like a chimney - practically setting his bed alight with every cigarette. However, underneath the almost pathetic exterior, as well as a lonely and deeply sad man was an intelligent, gentle man. Jim's bed was by a window, overlooking the playground of a school.

As I stood up after finishing the dressing, which we were there for, I saw a tear fall down Jim's cheek as he stared at the children running happily below him. My heart went out to him and yet I could not find any words to say. Here was a man with no 'life' as I would call it, and yet this was the way he had chosen to live. I began to feel angry with my mentor. Why didn't she do something about the situation? Put him in touch with organisations to help, etc.? But deep down I knew as well as she did, that this was the way Jim had chosen to live and we had no right to dictate our values to him.

As we were leaving, the tears still rolling down his cheeks, Jim said, with a touch of humour, "God, I'm a miserable old sod, aren't I?"

"Yes, Jim," said my district nurse, "but you can become very fond of miserable old sods sometimes, you know!" It seemed the perfect answer.'

Did you notice that this story began in the form of questions posed and answered by the student herself and ends with the magic moment of the humorous interaction between district nurse and patient, emphasising the connectedness of the relationship. The inclusion of Jamie's attention to detail in her story such as the 'tear rolling down his cheek' as he watched children playing in the playground (full of life as compared with him with 'no life') helps explain why her 'heart went out to him'. This shows the value of using detailed descriptions in your reflections. Jamie's attention to detail in her written reflection helps us to gain valuable insights into the patient's world. If we try to understand the story from her perspective, she is questioning whether people should 'be allowed' to live in a way which is risky and undesirable - an ethical dilemma. Her initial impulse was to say, 'Take Jim out of all this and make things better', demonstrating how much she saw herself as a caring nurse. She reflected, however, on how she changed her mind and related this to the need to uphold personal choice (Jim therefore being 'allowed' to take an active rather than a passive role) and uncovering another way of valuing him and acknowledging his importance (another active role) by means of an appropriate humorous response from the district nurse. This 'caring' exchange, described as 'a perfect answer' denoting a positive, supportive and non-patronising attitude towards the patient, was an important opportunity of learning for Jamie. She recognised this through her reflection and this is likely to influence her practice in the future.

In spite of the less than ideal circumstances, the positive exchange between Jamie's mentor and Jim is likely to have contributed to a connected and mutual relationship. Jim could easily have been seen as an unequal partner in this relationship - his lifestyle was unhealthy and his behaviour could be seen as self-destructive. However, what was really apparent was that the nurse used the opportunity Jim provided in using wry humour to sum up how he felt about himself by responding in a similar manner – a warm exchange from one human being to another. This is in line with Morse's description of a nurse–patient relationship which is built on reciprocity (a relationship in which one both gives to and receives from the other) and mutuality (a relationship based on shared trust and a feeling of affinity with the other).

Who is caring for whom?

From all this it follows that it may not be possible always to know who is benefiting most or even who is caring for whom. To illustrate this, Alex told of her experience as a patient in accident and emergency (A+E) after being knocked unconscious and suffering facial injuries following an unprovoked assault. Read her story and think about ways in which Alex was helping and supporting the student.

Case Study 2.3

'I was taken for a skull X-ray and a young student radiographer was left with me whilst the radiographers sorted out the equipment. After having several people around me all the time, I suddenly felt very lonely and when the student, trying to make conversation with me asked "How are you?" I burst into tears. The student looked very distressed and I realised that she must be feeling uncomfortable and probably didn't know what to say for the best. I didn't want her to feel like that so I tried to put her more at ease (and probably myself) by changing the subject. I said, "How long is your shift?" We chatted on about shift patterns for the few minutes which passed until the X-ray was ready to be taken.'

Many of these kinds of interactions occur all the time. You may have observed patients helping staff feel at ease (perhaps by initiating supportive conversations) and also patients sometimes do this with their relatives (perhaps trying to make them less worried by playing down unpleasant symptoms).

Another example of connectedness in the form of support, understanding and empathy is apparent in this next incident in which a nurse gave an account of her interaction with a family member. We think it is poignant in that, until a reflective workshop allowed her to explore the incident, the staff nurse who told the story overlooked the 'gift' she was given because she was distressed at her own perceptions of her inability to act in a supportive manner. When you look at the incident, think about significant features of the story in terms of how the newly qualified staff nurse was prepared for such an event and who helped her most.

Case Study 2.4

'A child had died on the early shift. I came onto the late shift with sister and a nursery nurse. I was a qualified nurse, but had no previous experience of a bereavement of a child. On the afternoon I was delegated to escort the child's grandparents to the Chapel of Rest to view their grandson. I was terrified and felt totally inadequate to cope with the grieving grandparents. I told sister this, but she informed me that I had to learn to cope with distressed relatives.

On walking to the Chapel of Rest I did not know what to say, so I kept quiet. On arrival I asked if they wanted to be alone, but grandmother insisted on me going in with her. I remember thinking to myself I have never seen a dead child before, and what will I do if the grandmother becomes hysterical? I felt totally useless and I must have looked it. I was taken by surprise when the grandmother took hold of my hand and said, "We will support each other dear."'

You should notice that the nurse says that she had no previous experience of bereavement of a child. She says that she was terrified and felt totally unable to cope with the grieving grandparents. The sister's reaction that she had to learn to cope would not have diminished her feelings of fear and inadequacy. As an experienced nurse, the sister was in a position to reassure and advise, and perhaps you will think it should have been part of the staff nurse's preceptorship or induction programme but it was the grandmother who took on the supportive role.

Why was the staff nurse 'terrified'? Perhaps she was reflecting her own fears related to the death of a child and felt that the relatives, would be unable to cope and she would have to bear the responsibility of dealing with this. Despite her fears and perceived deficiencies in caring for the grieving grandparents, she still went with the grandparents to the chapel of rest, and kept quiet when not knowing what to say. We know that many of us are fearful of silence, eager to fill it with sound of some sort. However, words can be inadequate in some situations and silence can be a significant feature of 'connected' relationships particularly if combined with appropriate touch. It should therefore be seen as an important part of the giving process.

In return for this staff nurse's courage, the grandmother gave her a wonderful gift, when she took hold of her hand and said, 'We will support each other dear'. Both the grandmother and Alex, in the previous story, were empowered by the support they gave. Instead of being 'victims' of the circumstances in which they found themselves, for a moment they became equal partners able to contribute to another's well-being. It is in the interest of professional health carers to appreciate this kind of mutual support and recognise the benefits gained.

To think about

It would be useful to consider your own experience of this as you go about your everyday practice.

+ Identify and record examples of psychological support you have received from patients.
+ Reflect on whether you were able to acknowledge any reciprocal/mutual gifts of support.
+ When you have done this, consider whether this helps you to understand more the value of the emotional care you give to others.

You might like to keep this as part of your learning diary or portfolio.

Learning further from our relationships

People who have learned to live with chronic conditions can teach us a great deal if we only listen! One student nurse acknowledged the help she had from Jonah, a young man with paraplegia:

> *'A lesson I shall never forget is that Jonah taught me how to care for patients like him. He showed me how to prevent pressure sores. Early on in his hospitalisation, it happened to him and he didn't want it to happen to anyone else.'*

The knowledge and experience of people with long-term conditions has been recognised as an untapped resource. In 2001, the Department of Health (DoH) published *The Expert Patient: A new approach to chronic disease management for the twenty-first century*. This emphasised the need to draw on the experience, knowledge and coping skills of people with long-term conditions such as heart disease, stroke, cancer, arthritis, diabetes mellitus, asthma, mental illness, epilepsy and also help them towards self-management. An observation was made that health professionals often stated that 'my patient understands their disease better than I do' (DoH, 2001: 4). Most people with long-term conditions live within their own homes rather than in hospitals and this inevitably affects the kind of relationship they have with care providers. This will be discussed further in a later chapter but the focus on patients as experts has re-emphasised the importance of seeing each individual patient as a unique learning resource.

Learning from George

In spite of the emphasis in nursing education on the importance of work-based learning for personal and professional development, there is still a tendency to devalue and overlook how much can be learned from the most fundamental aspects of all care provision for every patient. This is illustrated by Ellie (a student nurse):

Case Study 2.5

'When I started my placement on the unit my mentor apologised for me being placed there, saying he was afraid it wasn't very 'cutting edge'. I am afraid that I also thought the same way because I had been so caught up with the advances in nursing and the technical skills that I had undervalued and had almost lost what I had once believed were important aspects of care.'

However, during Ellie's ward placement her reflections on her interactions with a patient, led her to think again about why she had wanted to nurse in the first instance and also explore the current ideas she had about what it meant to care:

'Before starting my nurse training I believed that people wanted to be a nurse because they wanted to 'care' about others. My first real experience of hospitals was through visiting my grandma who was admitted on a couple of occasions towards the end of her life. At every visit, on entering her side room there were things, I felt, that had been overlooked by staff. Her glasses would not be on or she would not have her teeth in; she had a hospital gown on when two of her own nightgowns were in the locker. On one occasion there was a plate of untouched sandwiches on the floor next to her chair and a cold cup of tea on the table over the bed, in which she had been left lying down. As she needed help with her mobility and was registered blind, I wondered how the staff thought she would manage to drink it. None of the nurses seemed to know anything about grandma - they had just started their shift. These were not big things and the nurses, no doubt short staffed, were busy with more important things. However, to a relative they conveyed a lack of care, "who was looking after her?"'

When Ellie was in a practice placement during her first year as a student nurse, she had an experience that made her feel uneasy. She found that feeding a patient was not as easy as she had thought earlier. She began to realise that these 'small things/simple tasks/caring skills' are in reality quite complex, and offer opportunities for learning. As you are reading her account of her experience with George jot down what she might have learned from this experience.

Case Study 2.6

'I was on an early shift in a placement, working with people who were severely mentally impaired. I was asked to wheel a resident into the dining room and to give him his breakfast. This was not an unusual request. It was part of the normal morning routine, getting people up, washed, dressed and taken for breakfast.

But this was George. I had never fed him breakfast before or any other meal. In fact I hadn't really been involved before with any aspect of his care. There were a few other residents at the unit I hadn't had much involvement with just because that was how it had worked out. But I was conscious of feeling glad that I wasn't involved with George.

George dribbled constantly. I knew he couldn't help it, but he was always dribbling. He used to put his hands in his mouth and so always had saliva on his hands. When people fed him if they didn't look away from him he would just sit with his mouth open and not eat. If anyone caught his eye, be it staff or other residents, he would open his mouth and food would fall out. I hated saliva. Of all the bodily 'fluidy mess' it was saliva I could not stand. And seeing people eat with their mouths open, seeing chewed up bits of food in their mouths and on their hands, it could honestly make me gag.

As I pushed George along the corridor it was all I could think about. I wasn't going to be able to do it. I was going to feel repulsed by this poor man and it was going to be obvious. Going into the dining room a health care assistant had just finished feeding one of the residents, I tried to catch her eye in the hope that she would send me off to get someone else up and feed George herself. But she didn't and I pushed George to the table. Someone in the kitchen put a bowl of cornflakes on the counter. "For George," they said. "Great!" I thought.

Milk seemed to pour out of his mouth and down his chin. I got up to get some paper roll to wipe it with. When I got back he had cornflakes all over his hands. I wiped them off and decided it would be best to wipe his mouth and hands after each spoonful. I got some more paper roll. We were halfway through the bowl before I realised that we were halfway through and I hadn't felt sick, I hadn't even pulled a face. He seemed a lot less messy than I thought.

Then I started to wonder if he was aware of not being able to control it and how much I would hate it if I were George. George leaned forward and put his hand on my knee leaving a patch of gooey cornflakes behind. I looked at him, he smiled, and I smiled back. I thought, "It's nothing that won't wash off."'

Compare your findings with those of Ellie. When Ellie first started to reflect on the incident she wanted to focus on why the encounter had made such an impact on her. She was surprised and puzzled when she realised the experience she had with George was related to her thoughts about her grandmother's care and what she believed about good care and her reasons for choosing nursing as a career.

Reflecting on her experience had increased her self-awareness and prompted her to re-examine core personal values. Jones's (2004) use of the psychodynamic notion of transference might have helped her to understand the complexities of nursing relationships. In this, patterns of relating to others are influenced by our experiences of past relationships. This can be positive (as in Ellie's case because it may have helped her to see George as a person, just as she had seen her grandmother when she was dependent on others, although it was a very different kind of relationship) but there is also the potential for relational difficulties if we project on to others negative feelings we have within ourselves. Ellie reflects in the next case study.

Case Study 2.7

'Through reflecting on the incident, I believe that I had projected my dislike of saliva on to George as a person. This helps explain why I had avoided contact with him. Whilst I was disappointed in myself for discovering this, in retrospect I was grateful the incident had occurred, as I was able to become more self-aware with regard to my feelings and subsequent behaviour.

Also, because of my nurse training, I knew that nursing skills involved procedures such as giving injections, setting up drips and carrying out observations such as blood pressures. My reflections helped me discover that I had started to consider that feeding a patient was not particularly a 'nursing skill' that had required a deal of expertise and knowledge. After all, I had assisted my Grandma with her meals before undertaking any nurse training!

My feelings when involved with George were different from my feelings when caring for my Grandma, and at first I therefore did not recognise this involvement as caring. I had found it easy to care for my Grandma as I had an emotional bond with her. Caring for a stranger I discovered was not quite as easy.

One of my limitations was my aversion to saliva and I was put in a position that forced me to feed George. How I felt was incongruent with how I behaved, and I was conscious of the possibility that the inner self would betray the outer self. I feel I was eventually able to recognise I was caring for George because I fulfilled the task of feeding him. I paid attention to the little things, by wiping his mouth and hands during and after breakfast. I began to imagine how I would feel if I was in his situation and, by the end of the incident, I felt much empathy towards George.'

What else Ellie learned from the incident

Ellie found the incident helped her to consider many other aspects for which she needed literature to expand her knowledge and understanding:

'Looking at the literature on feeding I discovered that patients with dementia do experience feeding difficulties which change as the condition progresses These difficulties range from the refusal to eat, turning the head away, keeping the mouth closed, spitting out food to leaving the mouth open and not swallowing. This links with George and with many other clients on the unit.'

This made her think again about the way in which she was feeding George and the type of food she was offering him. She also looked at a wider range of literature and other theories related to such topics as the psychosocial aspects of eating and drinking and of communication. She considered other concepts such as empathy and unpopularity and their relationship to the care she provided. The experience with George therefore contributed enormously to her learning and her future practice.

If we return to the incident an important factor, which you may have noted, was the smile George gave to Ellie. This was an additional 'reward' for Ellie, influenced how she felt and helped to reinforce the importance of the learning she had gained about herself and what it was to truly care.

Whilst Ellie was searching the literature, she may have come across a similar kind of incident recounted by Redwood (2004: 130) who was undertaking research into learning in practice. She observed a young nurse sitting by the bed of an elderly woman trying to give her a drink of water. Just as in the incident with George described above, the nurse looked tense and anxious as the task was not easy and resulted in water constantly dribbling down the patient's chin and some choking and coughing.

> *'The nurse then repositioned herself and slightly moved the patient's head. This small adjustment made feeding the patient much easier. She then learned to go with the patient's rhythm of breathing through the mouth, sipping a little water, breathing through the nose and swallowing, followed by a moment's rest. Not too long to tire her patient, nor too short to rush her. I saw the nurse relax her body and develop an ease as she was slowly feeding her patient. She then began to speak slowly to the woman who responded by opening her eyes and looking at her. They spoke little, but for some time both women were in an intimate dialogue with each other.'*

Once again, a task for someone had resulted in a key learning opportunity and a means of establishing 'connectedness'. For Redwood (2004: 131), it was an opportunity for learning too which would influence her own development as a nurse researcher:

> *'I left the ward and I felt myself to be very fortunate. I realised that I had just witnessed a new member of our profession learn the highly complex and deeply human skill of enabling another person to drink. What I had seen was nursing. And I began to ask questions again. How did she learn the skill of feeding a patient who struggled to breathe? What happened between her and the woman that enabled her to learn from her?*

Time to think back

What has the incident with George taught us?

+ We have found that there is a great opportunity to provide sensitive and highly complex nursing care in areas which are often regarded as requiring little skill or expertise and to learn from the people for whom we care.
+ We can expand our ability to care by increasing our knowledge base by using theory to help explain and guide our practice.
+ Detailed and honest descriptive accounts of our experiences such as Ellie's can act as a springboard for immense learning.

Nurses have needs too

In discussing nursing, Bray (1998) is very forceful in her view that helping others is not an altruistic or unselfish act. As we have seen, nurses have needs in their relationships with patients and there are mutual benefits to be gained. Bray (1998: 99) goes further to claim that we may be drawn to help others because of our own 'emotional wounds'. She points out the positive aspects of this. 'This is not necessarily a bad thing', she suggests, since 'it makes good psychic and economic sense to heal oneself whilst promoting healing in others'. She goes on to quote Skynner (1989) who emphasised that mental health professionals 'are the only people willing and able to sustain their very difficult task of caring for others' mental illness perhaps precisely *because* they are getting something from it psychologically, something which they have been unable to obtain in the normal course of their life'.

We bring with us to every care situation emotional baggage or wounds, and for Kate, a student nurse, these may well have influenced the ways in which she cared for others with similar problems to her mother. She noted the time when she became more self-aware of her perceptions of her mother who had long-term mental health problems. Her written reflections on a visit to her mother in hospital recall the moment this occurred:

Case Study 2.8

'Everyone realises my mam is sick and there will never be a cure but IT still gets me down at times. It's been happening since I was eight. ... The depression, the medication, the hospital etc. I can't remember the last time I never NOT worried about her.

I visited her the other day and she appeared a little better but not a lot. However, there was quite a weird moment between us that scared me to bits but I feel that it was meant to happen. I was sitting with her on her stiff hospital bed and whilst she was talking to me her voice seemed to settle into the background like an echo and I struggled to listen to her as I went back in time. She spiralled away from me and my mind began to burst with memories and thoughts of her when I was little – when I really looked up to her and wanted to be just like her. I adored the way she loved life and the people in it and how simultaneously everyone loved her back. I could picture her reassuring smile, warm eyes and the way she presented herself. She was a true lady and a perfect mother.

Suddenly my body overflowed with the sickening and abrupt sensation of shock with the mother I saw before me now. I couldn't make the link between when I was a child and that moment. I stared at her, wondering who she was and where she had gone. ... Lost within herself and saturated in drugs. I felt gutted and proud of her at the same time. Her soft voice with its depth of confusion flooded back to my senses and she was back on her bed next to me gripping my hands. All at once I realised that this too was my mother. ... I know that this will be probably seem abstract to you ... I feel as though my inner self has grown and left the last skin of longing behind, like a butterfly. I feel free – free from grudges and bitterness, free from the past and free from my old disappointed searching self. ...'

Mental illness may affect our ability to see people as people, and the strength of Kate's story for us is that it highlights how easy it is to forget the individual even if it's someone close to us, and only see the condition or the difficulties surrounding them. It also demonstrates how beneficial it is when we remember them as human beings like ourselves with all our strengths and imperfections.

We need to recognise that nurses in all health care settings gain potential benefits from acts of caring. We all carry with us learning behaviours influenced by previous experiences (positive as well as traumatic or hurtful) and so need to remind ourselves of the importance of developing self-awareness, perhaps by using reflection or by being able to engage in informal or formal support groups. In our working life, we must recognise and accept that we all have needs, and are affected by our perceptions of how colleagues and patients interact with us. However, we need to be vigilant that we take care not to give less to those who seem to give less to us, such as those who might be categorised as 'unpopular' patients or clients.

Implications for informal carers

We can see that the act of caring for someone is complex and even in undertaking this for those we love, we are not doing so entirely for unselfish motives (the notion of altruism) since, as we have argued, the act of caring is not only beneficial for the recipient of the care but has important benefits for the care-giver as well. Turner (2005) asks whether people ever act from altruistic or unselfish motives and the debate about whether altruistic behaviour exists has engaged academics such as philosophers, biologists and psychologists for a long time. This may seem a little abstract and remote for our everyday concerns but has practical and economic applications to health and social care.

To think about

+ Think back to what you have read about mutual benefits of care relationships. Does this have any relevance for informal carers?
+ What might make them go on providing care?
+ What might make them reluctant to continue?

Looking at research on this topic can help your considerations. Brouwer *et al.* (2005) found that almost half the informal care-givers they studied (from a sample of 950 respondents) derived positive benefits from providing care themselves and that on average their happiness levels would decline if this care was handed over to someone else. This is an important point as it is so easy for people requiring care to see themselves only as a burden to others. Perhaps this indicates that there is a need for more acknowledgement of what care receivers are able to give to care relationships. The researchers also came to the conclusion that being in control of the process of caring seems to be particularly important for informal carers since once the 'caring starts to take control of them' (Brouwer *et al.*, 2005: 97), the negative aspects outweigh the benefits. They therefore emphasised the need for assisting and supporting care-givers to retain the benefits of providing informal care and retaining their sense of control over the situation. As we know and you may have noted, some carers labelled euphemistically as 'informal' may be providing care in very difficult and challenging situations (e.g. caring for a child who has complex care needs such as a tracheotomy, or a young woman with challenging behaviour, an older parent with Alzheimer's disease) and may need a great deal of support and help if they are to continue.

The research findings have relevance for us and need to be taken into consideration if we are to work effectively with patients and their families. We know that many families want to care for their loved ones at home but we need to help them feel empowered to do this so that they are in control of the situation rather than overwhelmed. Developing supportive relationships with informal carers is such an essential part of effective nursing care that we will revisit this important topic in more detail in Chapter 5.

Summary

In this chapter we have discovered, amongst other things, that:

+ Partnerships in nursing care can be very rewarding to both nurse and patient - it is a process of giving and receiving. Caring for others is connected with benefits to ourselves - one of mutuality and reciprocity.
+ There is a need to be aware of and accept emotional gifts from others. If we want to achieve true partnerships with patients we also have to acknowledge and value their contribution to our personal and professional growth.
+ Analysing our detailed reflections and using theory can help us gain more understanding of what it means to care,
+ It is important to help informal carers to maintain rewarding relationships with those for whom they care and we have to assist and support them so that they retain the benefits of providing care.

Looking forward

As you will see, we have collected additional caring indicators at the end of this chapter. These will be incorporated into our framework of caring at the end of the book. In the next chapter, in order to find out more about caring, we will use stories which focus on perceived inadequacies in care. These are important if we are to avoid difficulties and continue to develop caring relationships.

Activity

+ When you next go into practice, pay particular attention to communication exchanges which work well for both patient (and/or relatives) and you (or a colleague).
+ It might be useful to make a detailed note of such exchanges so you can reflect on why a particular exchange was mutually beneficial.
+ Consider how your reflections can help you towards providing evidence for some the outcomes and proficiencies set out in your nursing programme.

Caring indicators

1. Recognising what we gain and what we receive in relationships
2. Looking for opportunities to establish connectedness in relationships
3. Commitment demonstrated by giving time and identifying and acting on helping opportunities
4. Overcoming barriers in one-sided relationships
5. Seeing people as people not as problems
6. Sensitivity and responsiveness to details and minute or covert signals
7. Acceptance of emotional gifts and appreciating the benefits gained
8. Ability and openness to learn from patients
9. Assisting and supporting care-givers to retain the benefits of providing informal care
10. The importance of mutually beneficial communication exchanges, including the effective use of humour and silence

References

Barker, P and Davidson, B (1998) The heart of the ethical matter. In Barker, B and Davidson, B (eds) *Ethical Strife*. London: Edward Arnold.

Benner, P (1984) *From Novice to Expert: Excellence and power in clinical nursing practice*. Menlo Park CA: Addison-Wesley.

Bray, J (1998) Psychiatric nursing and the myth of altruism. In Barker, P and Davidson, B (eds) *Ethical Stride*. London Arnold.

Brouwer, W , Van Excel, N A J, Van den Berg, B, Van den Bos, G A M, Koopmanschap, M A (2005) Process utility from providing informal care: the benefit of caring. *Health Policy* **74**, 85-99.

DoH (Department of Health) (2001) *The Expert Patient: A new approach to chronic disease management for the twenty-first century*. London: The Stationery Office.

Jones, A C (2004) Transference, counter-transference and repetition: some implications for nursing practice. *Journal of Clinical Nursing* **14**, 1177-1184.

Lindow, V (1996) What we want from community psychiatric nurses. In Read, J and Reynolds, J (eds) *Speaking our Minds: an anthology*. Basingstoke: Macmillan .

Morse, J M ((1991) Negotiating commitment and involvement in the nurse-patient relationship. *Journal of Advanced Nursing* **16**, 455-468.

Roach, M S (2002) *Caring, the Human Mode of Being* (2nd edn). Ottawa, Ontario: CHA Press.

Redwood, S (2004) Case study 3: Careers in nursing research. In Freshwater, D and Bishop, V (eds) *Nursing Research in Context. Appreciation, application and professional development*. Basingstoke: Palgrave Macmillan.

Thomson, S (2005) Magic moments. *Nursing Standard* **19**, 70-71.

Turner, D D (2005) Altruism - is it still an anomaly? *Trends in Cognitive Sciences* **9**, 317-318.

Chapter 3
Putting the caring into care

LEARNING OBJECTIVES

By the end of this chapter you should have an understanding of:

1. How to recognise distress by 'tuning in' to the patient and their lived experience of care

2. How to increase skills in empathy and to see what interventions are helpful and what are not

3. The importance of effective reassurance

4. Behaviour by health care professionals which may result in loss of a patient's dignity

5. The impact of small acts of kindness

6. The benefits and contributions that expert patients can make to care

Introduction

In this chapter we will consider the impact of stressful or unhelpful interactions and interventions on service users and their families. Their stories will help us to consider situations in which nurses or other health care professionals may not have been intentionally hurtful but nevertheless have caused tension, suspicion, distrust and distress. As nurses, we need to face up to such situations and see what we can learn from them so that we will become more aware of such experiences and consider how we might better promote respect and dignity for the individual.

Not waving but drowning

We have included some incidents in this chapter which are traumatic and distressful because, unfortunate as they are, we need to face up to difficult situations and see ways in which we can avoid such situations in the future and enhance our practice. User perspectives are particularly useful as a means of uncovering deficiencies in care, helping us to increase skills in empathy and to see which interventions are helpful and which are not. Consider the following, written by Joanne who reflected on her postoperative experience and think about whether the nurse helped her to feel safe.

Case Study 3.1

'I had a tracheotomy tube in and not able to breathe properly. My mouth was swollen and I was gasping for air. I was trying to get the nurse's attention as she was at the foot of the bed, not looking at me. She was fiddling around with the charts writing down my saturation levels.

I wrote 'I can't breathe'.

"Well," she said, "you are 100% saturated with oxygen."

I wrote 'Yes, but I can't breathe'.

This happened three times. I wanted an explanation, but she continued to stand at the bottom of the bed working on the sats. Then I noticed my husband, Dave, was there and he asked me, "What is the matter?"

I pointed at the nurse and made a fist. Here I was, three hours out of surgery and I wanted to bop somebody. Dave held on to my hand and said, "You're something else, you are!"

Because the nurse who had looked after me earlier had made me feel so good and cared for and calmed me, I was upset that the second didn't see my distress. It wound me up completely.'

To think about

+ Think about what we can learn from Joanne's story about reassurance.
+ Think about a situation in your own practice where you or someone else has given a patient or their relatives 'reassurance'. Writing it down and reflecting (perhaps through the use of theory) will help you to unpick the characteristics of effective reassurance. Then read the next discussion to see how your findings match with ours.

You might like to keep this as part of your reflective learning diary or ongoing assessment record.

Reassurance is a word which, as nurses, we often use but perhaps don't think enough about what it actually means. Teasdale (1995: 79) saw it as 'an attempt to communicate with people who are anxious, worried or distressed with the intention of inducing them to predict that they are safe or safer than they presently believe or fear.' To do this we must first listen to someone, acknowledge their fears and take care not to respond in an overoptimistic or patronising way. Wynne-Jones (2006), who works as a GP, not only highlights the importance of reassurance to reduce anxieties but interestingly she recognised other advantages of this in making her job easier in terms of reducing repeated questions and consultations. She suggested five stages in the process of effective reassurance which you may find helpful:

+ eliciting ideas, concerns and expectations (she calls these ICEs);
+ checking and summarising these (this is a form of acknowledgement);
+ explaining what is happening and what can be achieved;
+ checking understanding;
+ entering into an agreement about a plan of action.

In Joanne's case, the nurse appeared to listen but she did not acknowledge her feelings. She looked for physiological evidence, significant as it was, but failed to take into account other important evidence – Joanne's fears and feelings. She therefore did not provide reassurance and evoke the calmness the first nurse had managed to obtain. She followed her own agenda, concentrating on the machine, and making Joanne feel that what she was saying was inconsequential. Joanne did not feel safe and therefore was not reassured.

Literature provides support for the view that Joanne is not alone in this kind of experience. Davies (2007) highlighted the significant number of intubated patients in intensive care units who have panic attacks and stressed the importance of constant reassurance by the nurse to minimise the symptoms.

In the rush and bustle of a busy day at work it is all too easy to miss that first important step in reassurance and see people as objects to be processed rather than individuals and therefore miss, ignore or misinterpret the signals of distress. Joanne's feelings of being misunderstood and her anxiety unrecognised reminds us of a poem by Stevie Smith (1981: 131), reproduced with permission entitled 'Not Waving But Drowning' which begins:

> Nobody heard him, the dead man,
> But still he lay moaning:
> I was much further out than you thought
> And not waving but drowning.

Joanne thought she was 'drowning' and the nurse did not allay that fear. She was able to contrast this with the previous care she had received where her perception was not based on the nurse using higher technical skills or knowledge but instead a caring and empathetic approach.

Using empathy

Empathy is often defined as the ability to put oneself in another person's shoes and is described by Rogers (1991) as the basic requirement for 'seeing' and 'hearing' in client-centred approaches. However, Skidmore (2005) also points out the uniqueness of every experience and he refers to Buber (1958) who argues that at best we can only gain a perception of someone else's experience. He suggests that we share 'affective resonance' but not the shared history, so every experience of emotional pain/trauma is unique to that person. It would appear that, for Joanne, the first nurse who cared for her had developed 'affective resonance' but the second had not.

Sometimes our deficiencies are inadvertent rather than deliberately cruel or unsympathetic but only by reflecting on examples of situations will we become aware of what people have found distressing and so will we be able to have greater insight into our own behaviour and the impact we might have on others. Developing empathy is therefore an ongoing learning process.

It may be seemingly minor incidents which have a great significance for participants and require empathetic exchanges. Esther described how anxious she was visiting her husband who had just been admitted to a trauma unit following a road accident. She approached a staff nurse who was standing at a notes trolley to ask how her husband was and what was likely to happen next. The staff nurse did not look up from the trolley but continued to look through the notes, saying 'He's OK – we'll know more when the doctors do their round tomorrow.'

Although this incident might seem insignificant and the response adequate, the lack of the small act of looking up and maintaining eye contact meant that Esther came away with the perception that the staff nurse was uncaring and did not realise the importance of the information she had been asked to give. It also left Esther with suspicions about the quality of care which was likely to be provided for her husband.

Personal evaluations of services will be particularly significant in the future if care is to be more personalised and responsive (Department of Health, 2007). Esther said her experience made her feel 'invisible' and powerless and many others have reported feeling this way, particularly older people. Theory can help explain this in a different way.

You may have come across the sociologist Goffman (1969) who has suggested that context influences the 'roles' we play in life. In this case, Esther seems almost a 'non-person' – her perceived role not important enough to engage in significant interaction. Buber (1958) an influential philosopher, has written about different ways we relate to others which may help us to understand Esther's perception. He talks about 'I – Thou' and 'I – It' relationships. It is only when we truly relate to another that we enter into an 'I – Thou' relationship , everything else he considers can be regarded as 'I – It' relationships – we regard others as we would objects.

We can draw parallels for this in the staff nurse's exchange with Esther. Without providing eye contact, warmth or interest, it became an 'I – it' encounter rather than an 'I – Thou'. It is important to remember that even brief exchanges like this can have an enormous influence on the way service users and their families perceive the care received.

Time to think back

Empathy is an important concept and you might want to think back on your own personal experiences where you felt that someone had become very close to understanding and entering 'your world' and because of this was able to help you in some way. You could also contrast this with an experience where you were not able to convey your needs and felt like a 'non-person' even if it was for a brief period of time. Understanding your own reactions to situations will help you empathise with others.

Dignity and respect

The importance of recognising needs and maintaining dignity and respect for older people is highlighted in the Philip Report undertaken for the Department of Health (2006) *Next Steps in Implementing the National Service Frameworks for Older People*. The report refers to the number of high-profile cases of poor treatment in mental health and general hospitals, in care homes and domiciliary care. 'Our definition of dignity is based on the moral requirement to respect all human beings, irrespective of any condition they may suffer from' (Department of Health, 2006: 4). The appointment of key nurses was proposed to ensure that older patients are treated with dignity and respect.

Whilst we would argue that this is an important strategy to protect the interests of vulnerable people, we see this as an indicator of failure – that the importance, value and impact of caring approaches have not been understood, measured or given enough attention in everyday practice whether in hospital or community care situations. It seems that it is often only when caring is missing at such a high level that it is noticed by the public and the press that it becomes the focus for discussion and action.

Consider the following story told by Miriam and jot down all the inadequacies in the care provided.

Case Study 3.2

'My Mum had a stroke two years ago but after a while, because she's so independent, she managed to continue living on her own with the family popping in regularly to help her out when she needed it. Unfortunately not long ago she had a lingering chest infection and when she developed chest pain, she was admitted to hospital. She's in her eighties so we were really worried about her as she seemed so frail. We were really upset to see her getting weaker very quickly and the lady in the next bed said that she wasn't eating at all but her meals were often taken away as nobody came to help her. She herself had mentioned it to the nurses and one came to help with the next meal but since then they seem to have forgotten that she needed help.

I was also upset to find that my mother was now incontinent and one day she started to cry and told me that the night nurses had told her off for wetting the bed. I didn't know what to do for the best but at least I thought I could make sure she was fed so I asked permission to come in at meal times and help my Mum and the sister said this would be very helpful as they were so short staffed.

One morning I was helping Mum with her breakfast. As I sat feeding her, Mrs Jones (in the bed opposite) rang the buzzer and asked to go to the toilet. The nursing assistant said, "Can't you wait till after breakfast Betty?" Mrs Jones said she was desperate so the nurse went for help and two of them, rather crossly, got her out of the bed and took her on a chair to the toilet. They hadn't covered her up properly and so her bottom was on full view to the rest of the room.

Later I overheard the two nursing assistants washing another old lady (behind the screens). What really horrified me was that it was obvious they were not talking to the patient but were discussing in great detail their escapades from their night out. I was embarrassed – and I consider myself broadminded! Their discussions shocked me. So much for care – I was really glad to take my mother home.'

Compare your findings with ours

We found that there were many faults in the care provided, such as there was not enough assistance from staff to ensure Miriam's mother's nutritional needs were met. This reflects findings by Age Concern (2006: 4) that 'One of the most frequent issues raised with Age Concern by the relatives of older people who have been in hospital is the lack of appropriate food and absence of help with eating and drinking for people who are unable to manage this for themselves.' Their campaign 'Hungry to be heard' set out seven steps to reduce the risk of malnourishment of older people when in hospital (you can find these by accessing the Age Concern website at www.ageconcern.org.uk/).

Being told off for wetting the bed would have made Miriam's mother feel embarrassed and that she was regarded rather like a naughty child. This would make her feel undignified, would have affected her self-esteem and showed a complete lack of respect and acknowledgement of her needs. Her incontinence could be a result of a general lack of care and attention. The way staff regarded toileting needs as an 'inconvenience' could also be seen in the way they responded to Mrs Jones's request. This was an uncaring approach.

Miriam might have found it difficult to complain about the service because of concern about how the staff might see her as a troublemaker and she might have thought a complaint could affect the care provided for her mother. There is the Patient Advice and Liaison Service (PALS) which can help people like her. This service was created to provide on-the-spot help in every NHS Trust by listening to patients' and families' concerns, identifying gaps in services and acting as a catalyst for change. In Miriam's case, PALS could also have given advice about the complaints procedure.

Staff called Mrs Jones 'Betty' – they would have needed to ensure that this was the name that she wished to be called. Otherwise they could be being overfamiliar and treating her again with disrespect. In addition, Mrs Jones was taken to the toilet inadequately covered. This showed disrespect and lack of understanding of Mrs Jones's needs for privacy and dignity. It would also have affected the way other patients in the ward thought they were regarded.

Staff were ignoring a patient whilst giving her intimate care. Their focus was themselves and their own preoccupations rather than the person receiving the care. It was also insulting to both the individual and all the other people in the room as they were overhearing inappropriate and embarrassing comments. This was truly uncaring care.

It is our contention that there is a need to become aware of situations such as Miriam has provided and to look at ways in which we can improve care for all patients, to ensure we do not engage in discriminatory practice, particularly towards those who are vulnerable such as older people, those in long-term care, those with learning disabilities, mental health problems and children. It should also be remembered that one of the most important ways of conveying respect and therefore promoting dignity is through effective and sensitive communication (Price, 2004).

Forgetting to ask what is needed

One way in which we can improve care is by working in closer partnership with patients and their families. As we have seen, attention, to both the artistry and the science of care, is necessary to give effective holistic care. We may be so engrossed in the tasks which are evident that we may forget to ask what is needed. A similar experience to Miriam's was identified by West (2006: 29), a nursing student who, as a result of her experience when visiting a friend (a patient in her seventies), realised the importance of proactive care.

> 'She was so quiet and unlikely to ask for help that I was worried that she had just been left. She was in pain but would not ask for relief – how could she when she was unable to see the call button? She was thirsty, but no one had thought to pour her a drink and place it within her reach. ... The ward nurses were not bad nurses – they were happy to help whenever I asked, but what this enough?'

It may well be quiet and compliant patients who may not gain the care they need because we are not adequately assessing them. Proactive interventions are an essential part of the caring process and these may be the result of assessment based on overt cues (signs of distress, dehydration, breathlessness etc.) as well as a result of asking the patient and/or their relatives what they need. In the rush and bustle of ward routines and procedures and even in a limited amount of time available to make a community visit, something obvious can easily be missed or assumptions can be made.

Consider the next scenario which highlights the importance of recognising the dangers of making assumptions and drawing inappropriate conclusions, sometimes transferred to others within a handover report.

Case Study 3.3

'The parents of a 9-month-old baby, who had been receiving chemotherapy on the ward, had just been told that he was not responding to treatment and nothing more could be done for him. They were given the option of staying in hospital or taking him home to die. The parents decided they would stay in hospital. I was on the late shift the day that this news was given to them and at the handover we were told that the family needed time to just be together and to keep nursing intervention to a minimum.

I felt worried about going into the room to give the baby his medication in case I upset the family. On entering the room, I was greeted as warmly as I always had been. The mother asked what was wrong as they had hardly seen anyone. I explained that the staff felt that they needed some privacy without nurses interrupting. This, I discovered, was not at all what they wanted and they felt abandoned by staff. They had elected to stay in hospital as they valued the support they had been given and wanted to continue as they felt it would make it easier for them to cope.

On reflection, I realised that the decision to give them privacy had been an assumption by my colleagues as to what the family wanted. I also wondered if it was a way of all of us being able to avoid a painful experience for ourselves. Put in a similar situation again, I realised I should try to negotiate what families really want, rather than try to assume their needs.'

You will have noticed from the above the nurse recognised that she and other members of staff, might have been avoiding the family almost unconsciously to lessen the distress they were also experiencing. We all do this and may resort to unconscious avoidance measures and overlook personal needs.

Other factors may influence our tendency to make assumptions. Claire told us of her experience when Penny, her 10-year-old daughter with severe learning disabilities, went into hospital. Penny uses sign language to communicate. It is not Makaton, but her own modified version because she has poor 'fine motor movements' so is unable to use her fingertips appropriately.

Case Study 3.4

'You have to really know Penny to be able to read what she is signing. She also conveys a lot with her facial expressions and eye moments. To someone else these are easily missed because they are so subtle. If we are not with her, she cannot communicate. When she went into hospital, she was signing 'drink' and the nurses did not understand. Fortunately we were there so we knew. There are other things – all of her food and drink has to be tepid, otherwise she will spit it out, looking as if we are trying to poison her. Without knowing her, the individual cannot care for her. Her right arm has to go in first when we are dressing her – this really matters to her. If one thing is not quite right, she refuses to do anything! Imagine not being able to tell people what you need, like the basics for life itself.'

To think about

+ Think of a practice situation in which you believe you have anticipated someone's needs and consider what evidence you used to come to that conclusion:
  - Did you follow a care plan?
  - Follow a role model?
  - Base your intervention on previous experience?
  - Look for verbal and non-verbal cues from the patient, relatives
  - Use observational charts?
+ You will have learned many ways to assess patients' needs, all of which are important and add to the overall picture. Has this chapter made you think again about the importance of asking the patient or their relatives how they view their needs?
+ Consider whether we are always able to meet these expressed needs or whether we have to sometimes use other strategies such as realistic but empathetic negotiation.

You might like to keep this as part of your reflective learning diary or ongoing assessment record.

Using patient experience

Listening to stories from patients and their relatives helps us to understand their lived experience and therefore recognise ways we might help. Warne and McAndrew (2005) stress that seeing patients as experts in their personal and cultural background and in the story of their illness can help maintain identity and lead to an exchange of important information and knowledge on the part of both patient and nurse. Each has an important part to play in this. 'Patient experience knowledge is different from the knowledge that is gained in grounding theoretical knowledge or practice knowledge – but it is part of both. … Patient experience knowledge requires the nurse to move their gaze from the body (as an object of intervention) to the person living a life' (Warne and McAndrew, 2005: 17). This way, they claim, nurses may better understand non-cooperative behaviour, non-compliance and the meaning interventions have for the patients.

Angelica had had a number of radical operations and extensive radiotherapy after she was found to have adenocarcinoma of her tongue base. The surgical procedures involved removal of a significant part of her mouth, tongue, salivary glands and the nodes around her neck. Also, because she had to have her tongue removed, she was given an operation that took part of her muscle from her lower shoulder to make her a new tongue. Angelica had speech therapy and had to learn to eat again. Her account of her everyday life helps us to see her as an individual – a young woman still trying to lead as normal a life as possible but whose needs have changed dramatically. Think about how the nurses might have met Angelica's need to communicate.

Case Study 3.5

'The social side of my life, the quality of life I have now has changed. ... I can't even have a normal meal with my friends because of my having to have peg feeds. ... And, because I can't speak properly, some people act as if they think that there is something wrong with me mentally. But I do go out and join in. I eat the soup, although it takes me forever. For instance, recently my friends and I were having a meal in a restaurant and we were having a good time. I had a mouthful of soup. There was something funny I wanted to say but, because it takes me ages to even eat soup, it was about five minutes before I managed to swallow it. When I had my mouth empty the moment was gone for my punch line – it was not funny anymore.

The same kind of thing had happened to me in hospital. The nurses always seemed too busy and I was often desperate to tell them something important but it took so long to get it out that often the moment was lost.'

Finding time

We think Angelica's story stresses that even if we're very busy it is important to find time to give patients the opportunity to communicate and therefore we need to find ways of enabling them to make their feelings and needs known. Parker (1999) highlights the problems of intubated patients in Intensive care units who, like Angelica, experienced distress related to their inability to release emotional tension and gain comfort through conversation. Her study also indicated that they were often not consulted about their care and they 'felt as though they were alone in a world removed from the world of others'(Parker 1999: 65). Not only is empathetic communication beneficial in terms of showing kindness and concern but it may well ensure less time is needed in future to calm distressed patients. Parker (1999) described how frightened patients could sometimes panic and react violently by pulling out tubes, lashing out or trying to get out of bed.

If we are proactive, looking ahead rather than reacting to situations as they occur, patients will feel that we respect them and want to help. In Parker's study, patients most often remembered staff with particular characteristics – those who were competent, kind, showed empathy and conscientiousness. Making sure that people do not feel neglected, even in hectic periods, is important and many nurses do this by renegotiating when they will be able to spend time with them. It is often these small actions that make people feel not forgotten.

Simple acts of kindness

Stories from patients also help illustrate the importance of simple acts of kindness and Georgina wrote.

Case Study 3.6

'I had just come back from the operating theatre and the nurse was lovely. Everything was hazy probably because of the morphine. I am not sure of the time but I don't think I had been back very long from the operating theatre. I sent my husband home. The nurse told me my mother rang. It was lovely to be contacted. The nurse washed me down and made me clean. I was intubated and ventilated so there was no way of communicating at the time except in writing.

She said, "I am going to get a mirror." I had the option to look. I could have said no. But I did and that was good. This got it into my head that I hadn't changed that much. I think it was being touched that made me feel human and accepted. That was a calming period and I slept.'

For patients such as Georgina, the need to maintain one's identity is particularly important and as professionals we may forget what aspects may have an impact on this such as, being touched and reassured in small ways, being kept clean, being involved in small decisions, receiving information such as calls from family and the reassurance of a recognisable self-image. This is reinforced by Magyar who gave this account of how she felt about a change to her appearance.

Case Study 3.7

'I had gone into hospital for one operation that should have taken me about one week to recover but I was in for four weeks. Before I was admitted I had planned to let my hair cover the scar on my neck so that it would not be so noticeable. They put about 4 or 5 elastic bands in my hair to tie it up before I went to theatre and my hair was put up into a paper hat. I had a bandage around my neck and tied at the top of my head. Like in the cartoons. Eventually they took the bandage off and I had dried blood in my hair but I was pleased as I now thought I could wash my hair once I got home.

But my curly hair had grown around the elastic bands. Peter tried all one afternoon (at home) but couldn't manage. So, then the hairdresser tried, for example with olive oil. I was there in the hairdressers all day with my nasogastric tube and they tried very hard to give me some privacy. They finally had to cut my hair off. This broke my heart. I was inconsolable. Peter said, "I can't believe you would cry over this. Everything you have gone through ... the operation – you never complained, you never cried. And they cut your hair off and ...".'

We also saw an example of this in Chapter 1, with Alan Bennett's description of the effect of his mother's hair being washed and left uncombed and uncurled after admission to hospital, so that it 'stood round her head in a mad halo' making it difficult for him to see how she would ever return to her 'normal' self. For Magyar the cutting of her hair had a similar devastating effect. Perhaps had the nurses known about the effect of the bands they would have thought of another strategy.

Acts of unkindness or insensitivity can lead to non-compliance in treatment. You can see how this happened in Lauren's story.

Case Study 3.8

'Postoperatively, I had many complications including breathlessness and I needed oxygen for this. It was decided that I would need to use the C Pap machine. Instead of this being explained to me and introduced to me gradually, the mask was forced on to me, with someone sitting on my hands! Perhaps it is not surprising that I panicked and refused to have this on. I was very upset. I wanted to go home. The female doctor declared that I would not even make it to the door and told me that if I refused to have the machine on then she would intubate and I would be awake. I did feel that I could have been treated in a kindlier manner by the nursing staff and the female doctor.

Following this I was visited by a male doctor who explained how the C Pap machine worked and why I needed it. As a result of this I agreed to try again and I managed to keep the machine on as long as I could put it on myself and I knew it would be removed if I panicked.'

Relating to and working with Lauren, instead of using a confrontational approach, changed a difficult situation into a collaborative partnership with a more effective outcome for all. Many patients remember other small acts of kindness which have had great significance for them, including Sharon.

'There were two excellent nursing staff on the night shifts, they washed my hair, they laughed with me, and they were friendly and reassured me that they would not leave me when they realised I was terrified. But I cannot remember their names – however, I do know that I prayed every evening for these two to be on duty.'

The outcomes of simple acts of kindness are often hidden. The staff nurses referred to by Sharon may not have been aware of the therapeutic effect of their interactions. Sometimes somewhat casual interactions can produce quite dramatic changes, and health care professionals who are sensitively attuned can change a difficult encounter into a more congenial one. A student nurse wrote of his experiences in an accident and emergency department.

Case Study 3.9

'One afternoon a qualified nurse ran up the ward to ask for help with Mick, a patient. He was quite well known to us since many of the staff had experienced episodes of violence with him, so we all went immediately. Mick was standing in the side room swearing like a trooper. We all tried to calm him down but this did not work. His language got worse as he got more agitated and I found this the hardest part. If anyone I knew called me these names I would have walked away from them – but here I had to stay and try to help calm him down.

Bill, one of the health care assistants, remarked wryly, "This is just like being at a Sunderland versus Newcastle game." With that, Mick stopped and looked at Bill.

"Do you support Newcastle Mick?" Bill asked.

Mick replied, "F--- No! I don't watch rubbish. I support a proper team."

It was the breakthrough we had all been waiting for. A conversation about football ensued and helped defuse a difficult situation.'

The student identified how an almost 'throwaway' remark provided the stepping-off point for perceiving Mick as an individual with his own place and preferences in society rather than 'the violent man with a psychiatric history'.

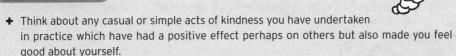

To think about

+ Think about any casual or simple acts of kindness you have undertaken in practice which have had a positive effect perhaps on others but also made you feel good about yourself.
+ Since it is easy to overlook these, next time you are in practice pay attention to (and perhaps record) them.

You might like to keep this information as part of your reflective learning diary or as evidence for your ongoing assessment record.

The effects of not paying attention

As we have said, we are not advocating a truly caring approach for humanistic reasons alone, important though these may be. If unthinking and ritualistic practices are followed, dire consequences may occur. Liam illustrates what can happen if something unexpected is not recognised and therefore not taken seriously:

Case Study 3.10

'I began to feel extremely hot every afternoon. I needed a fan and I kept saying, "I don't feel very well", "Do you think it is an infection?", "Do you think that is pus around the drain? It looks green to me". One senior staff nurse kept telling me over and over again that it was just oozing lymphatic fluid. My temperature, she said, was normal. But they only took it once a day on a morning. But I felt more and more ill – I felt faint and kept feeling as if I was passing out. I was too tired to protest further. My mother told me later that when she got home from visiting me she got on her knees and prayed, she was so worried about me. By the end of that week my mother, my partner and others could not believe how ill I was and were very worried because they did not have faith in what they were being told. They got together and managed to get the consultant in to look at me on the Saturday. I then got intravenous antibiotics and they removed the drains. The pus spurted out from the hole every time they dressed the wound. It was a severe infection.'

Liam who told us this story never wanted to go back to that particular hospital again; although other people will have different experiences, nothing could erase the fear and anguish he had in being disregarded. In some ways he was fortunate in that he had family and friends who were his advocates and played an important role in getting the care he required.

Partnerships in care – who knows best?

We must recognise that family and friends may find it difficult to get through the covert or hidden power that professionals and organisations hold and there may be problems in how they all work together to make decisions about the best care for the patient. Carol, a student nurse, expressed her concern about how staff, believing that they were doing the 'right' thing for the patient, deceived a relative who had a different view.

Case Study 3.11

'Fred is 70 years old and has suffered many strokes in his lifetime that have left him completely immobile, mute and victim of dementia. He is also blind. Joan, Fred's wife, lives in the home she shared with her husband before it became too difficult for her to care for him on her own. She comes to visit Fred once a day, having either lunch or tea with him. Joan has frequently expressed her wish to be involved in all aspects of Fred's care. She believes that in knowing him better than anyone else she is capable of standing in as his voice. ... A speech therapist visited Fred and expressed concern that one day he might choke. She advised that all of his meals were to be liquidised in order to reduce this risk. All staff agreed with this; however, Joan did not.

After listening to the speech therapist and almost every staff member explaining why it was a good idea, Joan calmly stated her point of view. She said that Fred had had a passion for food all of his life. He looked forward to mealtimes and as his health deteriorated this became one of his only pleasures. Joan said that she didn't expect any of us to understand but she knew her husband and what he would want. She told us that she couldn't give her husband much anymore but she could take a stand and make sure that at least he had nice food to eat. She added almost cynically, "if he dies choking, at least it will be something worth choking on - not just a pile of mush." The staff told Joan in no uncertain terms that they did not want to be responsible for Fred choking whilst one of them was feeding him. Joan said that she would take that responsibility as his next of kin and was willing to put it in writing.

The outcome was that when Joan was there, he was given solid food but when she wasn't the staff fed Fred liquidised food. Somehow I pacified myself with the thought that the staff were only doing it for Fred's own good, yet I knew in my heart that what we were doing was wrong.'

This is an example of an ethical dilemma related to risk management which happens every day in practice but in this case it was 'covered up' or 'managed'. The key issue for us in this story is the nature of true partnerships - if we are to work together with clients and their families an open and honest approach has to be used so that a solution based on mutual trust is found. Even if an intervention is perceived as being in the best interest of the patient, there is a danger of trust being shattered if the foundation for that trust is built on pretence.

Using guidelines and reports to inform practice

The NMC Code of Professional Conduct (2008: 2) recognises the importance of partnerships in care based on informed choice and the patient's right to decide whether or not to undergo any health care intervention. It states that 'Nurses must listen and respond to the concerns and preferences of people in their care.' Various government policies have also promoted patient choice and control over services (Department of Heath, 2001, 2005 and 2007) with autonomy and advocacy seen as key issues. However, as was explained earlier within *Guidelines for Mental Health and Learning Disabilities Nursing* (UKCC, 1998), these aspects need to be carefully considered so that mutually acceptable solutions to problems are arrived at. This may involve mediation with carers. The guidelines also recognised the difficulties inherent within the client-professional power balance. 'You must not practise in a way which assumes that only you know what is best for a client. This may create dependency, hinders team work and can interfere with the client's right to choose. Some clients may be highly suggestible and thus more likely to agree to suggestions or choices from those in positions of authority. Advocacy is about promoting clients' rights to choose and empowering them to decide for themselves' (UKCC, 1998: 14).

Skidmore (2005) suggests that there is a place for the expert professional in giving advice but not to act as a 'life director'. 'The expert should use their expertise to facilitate another's journey; be it through health, education or the workplace. To do otherwise removes control from the individual and makes them forever dependent upon the 'expert' ' (Skidmore, 2005: 25).

People with learning disabilities may become particularly powerless because of the way they are perceived and this may have a disastrous effect on any care or treatment they receive. The *Treat Me Right!* report from Mencap in 2004 highlighted the unequal health care that they often receive from health care professionals and this was reiterated by the Disability Rights Commission in 2006 which published the results of a formal investigation into physical health inequalities experienced by people with learning disabilities and mental health problems. A Mencap report which followed on from this entitled *Death by Indifference* and published in 2007, claimed 'institutional discrimination' within the NHS and included case studies outlining the traumatic experiences of six people who died whilst in hospital care. A common complaint of their families was that they felt consistently ignored when they expressed their concerns. The report called for improved staff training to reduce the risk of diagnostic overshadowing which is explained as the belief that 'a presenting problem is a feature of someone's learning disability and that not much can be done about it' (Mencap, 2007: 20). As we have seen, nurses have an important role to play in listening to families and getting their help in recognising important, and perhaps to us uncommon, indications of problems. We need to be aware that family members or other carers can play a key role in interpreting distress cues and other signs and behaviour which might be missed by professional staff.

The need for anti-discriminatory practice

Although for people with learning disabilities there is a particular problem, there is also danger in letting our assumptions misinterpret important cues with other client groups. Some people have great insights into the way stock answers are sometimes used to 're-assure' patients and dismiss their concerns. Jasmin, a student nurse, told us how much she learned from Gordon, a 75-year-old man who asked a doctor, undertaking his ward round, to look at his very painful knee.

'Don't worry about it, ' the doctor said sympathetically; 'it's just old age.'

'Well,' said Gordon, 'the other knee's the same age but that isn't giving me any problem!'

We need to be very careful that we listen to what people are saying and that we do not discount it by interpreting it as entirely due to some pre-existing condition such as age or disability.

People with mental health problems sometimes face prejudice when accessing health services. Assumptions made about them may interfere with diagnosis but may more commonly be associated with reactions of indifference or frustration. Hilary, a student nurse, wrote of her concern about the way Jason was treated in an accident and emergency department. Consider and reflect on this account.

Case Study 3.12

'The paramedics brought in Jason who claimed he had taken forty-five co-codamol tablets with alcohol. They handed him over to my mentor who looked at Jason sitting in the corridor and said to me, "Do that man's observations please and take him to the assessment room" (this is where the psychological assessments are carried out). I was very shocked and confused by his attitude towards Jason. My mentor did not communicate with Jason at all, which was out of character for him. I walked over to Jason and explained I was going to take his temperature and blood pressure. As I was applying the cuff he began to cry. I did not know what to say to him and was worried in case I said the wrong thing and upset him further so I smiled sympathetically and touched him on the arm but I did not know whether that was the right thing to do or not. After I'd finished the observations I escorted him to the assessment room. I asked Jason if he was all right and if he wanted anything and then went back to inform my mentor about the observations I had taken. My mentor explained that Jason was a 'regular attender' at the A+E, often attending after taking an overdose. This seemed to anger my mentor. I could not understand why he felt this way as there must be a reason why Jason kept trying to commit suicide. I was shocked that, although he was treated for his overdose, no member of staff showed they cared about Jason or talked to him as a person. They seemed to be wanting to get him out of the A+E as quickly as possible.'

Time to think back

+ How would you describe the attitudes of the staff in the accident and emergency department?
+ How did these attitudes influence their behaviour towards Jason?
+ What effect did the experience have on Hilary?
+ Do you know of any theoretical perspectives, guidelines or reports which might have informed practice?

Compare your findings with ours

Jason's presence in A+E seems to have evoked strong feelings of anger and perhaps frustration. He was the subject of stereotyping by Hilary's mentor (a generalisation that he belonged to a group of 'regular attenders', seen as having certain characteristics). This stereotyping may have led to the belief that people who self-harmed 'wasted staff time' and were themselves to blame for their actions (negative prejudice). This may have resulted in discrimination, in that there may have been inappropriate or inadequate care for Jason. You may have thought that in this case the mentor demonstrated this by avoiding Jason's care and leaving it to Hilary who was inexperienced and finding it very difficult to know how best to communicate with him. She needed guidance and reassurance from a mentor who needed to review his own approach not only to Jason but also to Hilary, perhaps through gaining more guidance and support for himself. You may have in your reflections, psychological or sociological literature or nursing resources which have helped you to understand these key concepts in more depth.

You may have included guidelines from the National Institute for Clinical Excellence (NICE) which were developed in 2004 in response to the 'unacceptable' and sometimes punitive treatment of the large number of people who deliberately injure themselves. These guidelines emphasised the need for health care professionals to show compassion and understanding, take account of the likely distress associated with self-harm and ensure that people who self-harm are adequately assessed. They should be asked to explain their feelings and understandings in their own words, in a private and safe environment. The guidelines go on to say that 'In caring for people who repeatedly self-harm, health care professionals should be aware that the individual's reasons for self-harm may be different on each occasion and therefore each episode needs to be treated in its own right' (NICE, 2004: 8). In Jason's case the mentor did not seem willing to do this. However, there is also a recognition of the stress and demands of caring for people who self-harm. The report acknowledges that providing treatment and care for them is emotionally demanding and it suggests that all staff involved in this kind of work should have regular supervision so that they can explore its emotional impact on them. Hilary was surprised because the reaction to Jason by her mentor seemed out of character, so it seems likely that he needs support so that he has a chance to talk through his negativity and gain more understanding and guidance.

We have talked about the importance of empathy, but as we struggle with difficult situations, the need to be caring can make heavy demands on us. According to Salvage (2006: 22), this is not just being polite or superficially pleasant. 'The genuine empathy that generates compassionate action is creative and challenging, not the sugary sort of niceness so often linked with the traditional image of nursing.' This may be particularly challenging when people such as Jason present us with difficult problems for which we can see little solution. However, if we are to be truly caring, we need to find ways in which we contain our frustrations and misgivings and learn to work with them so that we can ease, rather than increase, their problems.

To do this we must be able to identify and learn to overcome the prejudices which are part of all of us. At times, these may be because of lack of knowledge or familiarity concerning people from a particular culture, for example black or ethnic minority groups. We may also make false assumptions and develop misunderstandings about people with particular conditions or histories, or those who belong to different religions, groups or backgrounds from us. These prejudices can lead to uncaring attitudes and behaviours and are against the NMC Code of Conduct (2008) which you should have included in your reflections since this is the code outlining standards for conduct, performance and ethics, under which we must all practice. For example, the code instructs us to make the care of people our first concern by treating them as individuals and respecting their dignity.

Working together

People with long-term conditions are also in particular need of good working relationships with health care professionals. The code of conduct highlights the importance of collaborating with those in our care. Recognition of the knowledge and skills of people with long-term conditions has been acknowledged by the Department of Health (2001) in its document entitled *The Expert Patient: A new approach to chronic disease management for the twenty-first century*. This report advocated a shift towards more equal partnerships between service users and professionals in working together and gaining more understanding about how people can best manage chronic conditions.

Creating a 'patient-led' NHS is a high priority, and within acute and community care settings the need for greater responsiveness to users needs and flexibility in the way in which care is provided is gaining greater momentum. In 2007, Gordon Brown, the prime minister, took this even further by calling for 'an NHS of the individual'. Many patients have extensive experience of a variety of hospitals and wards, making them 'experts' in evaluating what caring really means. If no one listens to patients with experience or their relatives or if they are too frightened to say what they really think of the care they receive, we will be unable to draw directly on this expertise. Toni, who has lived for years with chronic asthma, reflected on one of her admissions to a particular hospital in this way:

> *'I was frightened to say too much because of possible repercussions. ... I will never go back to that hospital. I believe they could have killed me – they didn't listen to what my husband said had helped before. I did not complain directly. But when the hospital posted me a questionnaire I completed it because I could remain anonymous.'*

Whether Toni was right or wrong in her criticisms is not the issue here. The point we are trying to make is that a culture of open dialogue must be created so any misconceptions can be clarified, fears reduced, assumptions challenged and immediate action taken when required. Stories or incidents from practice, particularly if they are apparently critical of care, are sometimes criticised for being individual perspectives and therefore may be considered not to be truly representative. However, we are suggesting that by using incidents such as those included above, much may be learned about how actions are perceived. Rolfe (2005) reminds us that although we must learn from patients, the patient's word is not 'a sacred text never to be challenged'. Realistically, people do make mistakes, are sometimes hard to communicate with or have particular behaviours or characteristics which we dislike or with which we disagree. However, Rolfe's view is that we must enter into a dialogue with them so that we understand their preoccupations and concerns and also, most importantly, try to help them to understand us. 'The patient experience is constructed and shaped through dialogue; it is only in the sharing of the experience that it is (trans)formed into knowledge' (Rolfe, 2005: xiii). We also think reflecting on distressing incidents told to us by patients will help us to gain self-understanding and free us from unthinking and discriminatory practices which will be perceived as uncaring.

Summary

In this chapter we have considered the need for putting more 'caring' into care. We have looked at both caring and uncaring moments in practice. The stories we have chosen of uncaring or negative attitudes may have not led to official complaints or investigations into professional misconduct but have been the kinds of events that can occur almost every day in practice and are mainly the result of unthinking or uninformed care rather than deliberate cruelty. Nevertheless, they can cause extreme distress and may have long-term effects on service users and their families. We have seen that to overcome such difficulties we need to focus on:

+ Developing a heightened awareness by listening to and 'hearing' patients' lived experiences.
+ Simple acts of kindness which may be easily overlooked, hidden and undervalued.

+ Developing and using skills of reassurance and empathy.
+ Being proactive about care needs.
+ Being aware of our own assumptions and promoting and engaging in anti-discriminatory practice.
+ Working in partnership, including acknowledging the contribution of the expert patient.

Looking forward

The impact of caring in terms of the nurse's emotional involvement cannot be underestimated, particularly given the unpredictable and sometimes distressing nature of nursing care. As we have seen in this chapter, there are situations which are challenging and require the expenditure of considerable emotional energy, sometimes known as 'labour'. These aspects and professional boundaries which need to be taken into account will be explored within the next chapter.

Activity

+ Reflect on your care and consider whether you have made assumptions about the people you have cared for.
+ Have you had to revise your views in the light of experience?
+ What has that taught you about your future practice?
+ Use the indicators below to see how they can help you to engage in anti-discriminatory, caring practice.

Caring indicators

1. Simple acts of kindness
2. Promoting dignity
3. Using and developing skills of empathy by 'tuning in' to the patient
4. Ability to move our gaze from the body (as an object of intervention) to the person (living a life)
5. Developing trust
6. Giving effective reassurance by giving the other person confidence in our ability to listen and to help them
7. Being proactive – asking patients what they need – not waiting to be asked
8. Recognising the limitations of one's skills
9. Entering into a partnership with patients and their families to gain knowledge and share the 'power'
10. Engaging in anti-discriminatory practice by respecting another human being, irrespective of age, gender, cultural origins, class, status or condition from which they suffer

References

Age Concern (2006) *Hungry to be Heard: The scandal of malnourished older people in hospital*. London: Age Concern.

Buber, M (1958) *I and Thou*. New York: Scribner.

Davies, D (2007) Reflection on practice: an intubated patient suffering panic attacks. *Nursing in Critical Care* **12**, 198-201.

Department of Health (2001) *The Expert Patient: A new approach to chronic disease management for the twenty-first century*. London: The Stationery Office.

Department of Health (2005) *Health Reform in England: Update and next steps*. London DoH.

Department of Health (2006) *Next Steps in Implementing the National Service Frameworks for Older People*. London: The Stationery Office.

Department of Health (2007) *Our NHS, Our Future*. Interim Report. London: The Stationery Office.

Disability Rights Commission (2006) *Equal Treatment: Closing the gap. A formal investigation into the physical health inequalities experienced by people with learning disabilities and/or mental health problems*. London Disability Rights Commission.

Goffman, E (1969) *The Presentation of Self in Everyday Life*. Harmondsworth: Penguin.

Mencap (2004) *Treat Me Right!* London: Mencap.

Mencap (2007) *Death by Indifference Report*. London: Mencap.

National Institute for Clinical Excellence (2004) *The short-term physical and psychological management and secondary prevention of self-harm in primary and secondary care*. Clinical Guidelines **16**. London: NICE. Accessible on www.nice.org.uk/ (last accessed (29 Oct. 2007).)

NMC (Nursing and Midwifery Council) (2008) *The Code: Standards of conduct, performance and ethics for nurses and midwives*. London: Nursing and Midwifery Council.

Parker, V (1999) On confronting life and death. In Madjar, I and Walton, J (eds) *Nursing and the Experience of Illness Phenomenology in Practice*. London: Routledge.

Price, B (2004) Demonstrating respect for patient dignity. *Nursing Standard* **19**, 45-51.

Rogers, C R (1991) *Client-centred Therapy*. London: Constable.

Rolfe, G (2005) Foreword. In Warne, T and McAndrew, S (eds) *Using Patient Experience in Nurse Education*. Basingstoke: Palgrave Macmillan.

Salvage, J (2006) It's the action that counts. *Nursing Standard* **20**, 20-23.

Skidmore, D (2005) The person as a life expert: this is not a love song. In Warne, T and McAndrew, S (eds) *Using Patient Experience in Nurse Education*. Basingstoke: Palgrave Macmillan.

Smith, Stevie (1981) Not waving but drowning. In Smith, S Collected Poems. New York: New Directions Publishing Corporation.

Teasdale, K (1995) Theoretical and practical considerations on the use of reassurance in the management of anxious patients. *Journal of Advanced Nursing* **22**, 79-86.

UKCC (UK Central Council for Nursing, Midwifery and Health Visiting) (1998) *Guidelines for Mental Health and Learning Disabilities Nursing*. London: UK Central Council for Nursing, Midwifery and Health Visiting.

Warne, T and McAndrew, S (eds) (2005) *Using Patient Experience in Nurse Education*. Basingstoke: Palgrave Macmillan.

West, L (2006) Student experiences in the real world of nursing. Starting out. *Nursing Standard* **20**, 29.

Wynne-Jones, M (2006) The patient who won't be reassured. *Pulse* **37**, 72.

Chapter 4
The emotional world of nursing

LEARNING OBJECTIVES

By the end of this chapter you should have an understanding of:

1. How emotions may affect your care in practice including your judgements and behaviour
2. Emotional labour as an essential part of caring
3. How identification with particular patients can affect our emotional balance
4. The parameters of the professional relationship
5. The importance of using opportunities for reflective learning

Introduction

In this chapter we will explore the emotional world of nursing. As nurses, whether qualified or students, we are often witness to traumatic, life-changing events and are also undertaking complex (and often undervalued) caring needs of vulnerable people with long-term disabilities. We need to respond quickly to acute and unpredictable situations and also to cope with everyday demands on us as we try to be physically and psychologically available to others. So nursing is far from an easy job.

Incidents and scenarios we have collected from our student nurse workshops indicate that, from the very beginning, it is important for students to explore the parameters, rules or boundaries of their work. The students' stories clearly show that they can be very uneasy about what it might mean to really care, how much emotional involvement there ought to be with clients and their families and how different types of emotional involvement (or otherwise) can affect themselves and their clients. Our students raised numerous questions about their concerns, for example: Should I attend the funerals of people I particularly care for? Where does my responsibility end? How should I feel about this? Am I a bad person if I don't get upset at something that others find harrowing? What am I to do with these guilty feelings? When I feel overwhelmed by events, should I try to shut off from emotional involvement? Why do I feel so guilty if I cannot give the amount of care I would like? These are just a few of the questions that caused anxiety for a large number of our student nurses. No doubt you will have felt uneasy about similar issues as well.

In this chapter we will explore some of these questions and again use stories to help us see the kinds of experiences that can have an emotional impact on nurses.

Caring for people – emotional work

Nursing is not just a series of tasks which have to be undertaken in a prescribed timeframe, although it may seem like this at times. Read Andy's story to see how a qualified mental health nurse reminded himself of the most important focus of his work.

Case Study 4.1

'As a community psychiatric nurse (CPN) for the older person I had a lot of new referrals to visit. It was a Monday morning and there had been a heavy snowfall the night before. I was very keen to start seeing these new clients, but had to see Terry, a 65-year-old. I noticed the path had been cleared. Thinking it was Terry who had done this, I called out "Who's been busy this morning then?" It was his brother. Terry had died that morning, clearing the path, due to a heart attack. I stayed and spoke to his family.

On leaving the village I saw a funeral car arriving at the home of a woman I had visited recently and who had then been admitted to the psychiatric hospital. She had died there but I had not been informed. I called to see the family.

Driving back, I reflected that earlier that morning I had felt 'bogged down' with the physical aspects of my work and the problems. The events of the morning brought it back to me that primarily I deal with, and get to know, people. I was not so hassled that week, reminding myself of this.'

Reflecting back on two unexpected deaths caused Andy to pause and review what his work was really about. His relationship with both patients' families prompted him to demonstrate a caring attitude and acknowledge the importance of their loss. Andy was an experienced nurse and was able to find his own particular way of effectively coping with any sadness he might have felt. He seems not to have become hardened to the death of his clients and saw his care of relatives as an important part of that care. Andy gave us this incident at a reflective workshop for qualified nurses, when he chose to look back at the importance of his feelings. Andy, like many nurses however experienced they are, find 'debriefing' (or talking over the situation with supportive others) beneficial after such an event. Parkinson (1997) argues that this helps to 'normalise' emotions, making individuals aware that their feelings are normal for what they have experienced. This is important since Smith (1992: 96) suggests that death and dying can call for 'the ultimate emotional labour'.

Linking theory to practice

You might have noticed that Andy said that he had been 'bogged down' with the physical aspects of his work. However, he realised the importance of the emotional side of his work in caring for people. In Chapter 1, we discussed the view that the demands of emotional work can be equally as hard as physical and technical labour. Sociologists such as Strauss *et al.* (1982) and James (1992) have emphasised the importance of taking this into account since it has implications for both carer and the person being cared for. They suggest that changes in modern medicine have led to a shift in emphasis from holistic regard for the individual to a biomedical model with a focus on the diagnosis and treatment of physiological malfunctioning of particular organs or systems. However, the success of modern health care in terms of the use of technology and a range of medical interventions and drugs, has meant an increase in the complexity of the care provided and in the skills required to do it. Such care has overshadowed and devalued emotional care although there is evidence of its increasing importance. Phillips (1996) sees this in terms of providing reassurance and support, not just to ensure compliance but also in helping the overall psychological and physical well-being of the patient. The effect of emotional labour on health care professionals was also recognised by James (1992) who saw it as difficult, personal, often upsetting and requiring a great deal of thought, skill and time.

Acknowledgement of the need to provide emotional support as part of holistic-centred care has been recognised in nursing in the promotion of individualised care plans, models of nursing and the named or primary nurse. In spite of all this however, the low status of emotional work may lead to unrealistic expectations and little support for a complex task. This could have adverse effects in the future.

In her study of student nurses' experiences, Smith (1992: 110) commented that there was 'an expectation that the more senior a student was the more likely she would be expected to cope with upsetting situations. It seemed that because students' feelings were rarely acknowledged in the open arena of the ward that they were likely to develop distancing strategies that kept them from personal involvement. They recognised that, as they progressed through their careers, they might become hard. But they also recognised that if they hardened and distanced too much they would be unable to nurse with feeling.' Reflection can help us to acknowledge and work with our feelings about events.

To think about

Think of an incident from practice and analyse it. We have chosen a framework developed by Smith and Russell (1991) which was slightly amended by Schutz, Angove and Sharp (2004: 58) to help you do this:

+ Write a description of the incident.
+ Outline why you chose the event and how and why it is significant for you.
+ Identify any key issues (perhaps questions which emerge) and why they are important.
+ Reflect on:
  - How you were involved, why and what you felt.
  - Why you behaved the way you did and how you made your decisions.
  - The part that others played and why you think they behaved as they did.
  - What else was happening in the context at the time?
  - The relevant theoretical background.
  - What action might be indicated either now or in the future?
  - How you evaluate what happened in terms of what you have learned in a specific and in a general sense.

You might like to keep this information as part of your reflective learning diary or portfolio.

Your analysis may have uncovered uncomfortable or confusing feelings. However, if you managed to work through the whole framework, including the use of theoretical resources, you may have found that this has helped you to clarify your thinking, emotions and perhaps your behaviour. It is not an easy task to be self-critical but you will find it can help to bring out the positive as well as the negative ways in which you respond to situations. The framework also points out that you should consider the effect of your reflections on your actions in the future. We all need to think critically about our practice in order to learn and develop from it. It is a never-ending quest throughout our professional lives so the skills you acquire now as a student will help you in the future.

Managing emotions

There is a need, if we want to be truly caring and effective, to find some sort of balance between being neither 'overemotional' nor blasé. The following stories give you an idea about some of the difficulties associated with managing feelings about an aspect which we may find particularly problematic – caring for the dying. They also demonstrate that an opportunity to discuss incidents and feelings with others is beneficial and supportive. Staff nurses at a mentor workshop noted that every experience of caring for dying patients and their relatives was unique and, even if expected, could result in vividly retained memories.

Case Study 4.2

'A lady died in the ward. My student had never seen a dead body before so I realised it was going to be hard. ... During the coffee break I took the opportunity to talk things over with her. There were a few of us who were talking about our experiences and we said, "Oh God, do you remember the first time we saw anybody die or have an arrest?" "Yes, I'll never forget the first woman I saw dead. Not that it was a horrible experience. It wasn't; just that's always going to stay with me."

I think a student is often facing new experiences and we had a particularly horrible death not so long ago. That is not a very nice way of putting it, but it was a stressful death for the few students that were around. ... A student had been there when the wife ran out of the room screaming as he arrested. So she basically got it 'full on'. I thought that it was really important for someone to go through that with her because the wife was still hysterical over an hour later. This guy was young!'

The above incidents show that the mentors were sensitive to the needs and feelings of students. They empathised with the students and used their own past experiences to help them. Being able to talk over events meant the staff were also able to consider their own feelings and reactions to the dying patients and their families. This is an example of the importance of passing on 'tacit' knowledge which is often hidden, or embedded, within nursing and which you may not find in your textbooks. In this case the mentors shared their knowledge and experiences of how to deal with such difficult situations in practice. They recognised the importance of helping students with the 'emotional labour' associated with death and this is important as it is likely to strike a chord within us, for example, regarding our own mortality and the transient nature of all human beings.

Connecting with a dying patient

Read the traumatic incident below written by a third year student nurse and consider why it was particularly emotional for her.

Case Study 4.3

'On a night shift we received a trauma call at approximately one in the morning. We were informed that we were to receive a young male with multiple stab wounds. In response we put out a trauma call. This requires a member from each discipline to attend A+E should their expertise be required, for instance anaesthetics, surgery, orthopaedics and the night sister. We prepared ourselves for the arrival of the patient, we wore apron and gloves, linked up the ambu bag to the oxygen, ran some fluid through ready and set up the trauma sheet and then we stood waiting.

On arrival of the young man, the paramedics instructed us that the most severe wounds were on his back but we soon realised that his puncture wounds were everywhere. He had a large slit from his mouth up his cheek, which was horrible. He also had puncture wounds to his arms and hands, probably from where he had lifted his hands to try to protect himself.

We immediately rolled him onto his side and took down the paramedic's dressing to assess the severity of the wounds to his back. There were three severe stab wounds to his back. The sister dressed them with a pressure dressing. Fluids were commenced and regular blood pressure results were monitored. He was conscious with a Glasgow Coma Score (GCS) of 15/15. He constantly asked for our names. With each new set of hands he felt touch him he asked who it was and what their name was. He was so grateful and kept saying "Thank you, if the paramedics hadn't got there when they did I would be dead now wouldn't I?"

He had an oxygen mask on but the doctors decided that he required chest drains. It was all happening so fast that I'm not sure why he needed them, whether it was because he wasn't saturating enough, or his chest wasn't rising properly or whether it was due to the area in his back that the stab wounds were I am honestly unsure. They decided to put bilateral chest drains in and whilst the left sided chest drain went in relatively easily, the doctor carrying out the right sided chest drain initially had some difficulty getting it in. They asked me to hold his hands while they put the chest drains in. This was probably partly for some reassurance, but also to literally hold his hands down to prevent him from pushing his hands up to stop the painful stimulus of inserting the drains. Even in pain he was much stronger than I was. I held his hand and he asked me my name, and said it was nice to meet me. I replied that it was nice to meet him too. He squeezed my hand and I squeezed his back. As I did so my finger seemed to disappear, it had sunk into one of the wounds in his hands. They were bleeding badly. Sister seemed to notice the blood loss at the same time as I did and I suggested we dress his hand. She agreed and held his hand up off the bed to enable me to dress it. He was transferred to theatre.

I had to go and attend to the rest of A+E, which was extremely busy. ... The department was packed and we had to continue attending to other patients but we all kept making comments about how we wondered how he was and informing each other of any news. It was a waiting game. Just before 7 a.m. the theatre staff came to retrieve his family. He was dying and they took them to be with him for his last few minutes. They escorted them to the recovery room. It was so horrible! I had a numb feeling afterwards. ...'

Case Study 4.4

Compare your considerations with part of the student's explanation of her feelings below. Note the way she uses theory to help her to do this.

'... It would be fair to say that I myself had become blasé in dealing with trauma situations as they had never affected me personally before. Rather interestingly Gibson and Iwaniec (2003) point out that the word trauma comes from the Greek and means to pierce or puncture armour. They state that it is important to consider this when preparing helpers to face incidents that have the potential for piercing their usual coping strategies. It is clear that my own coping strategies appear to have suffered a similar assault with regard to this incident.

The reasoning for my feeling so emotionally involved has still probably not been clarified. It was due to a number of reasons. The patient was about the same age as me. ... More importantly though was the fact that he knew my name and I had held his hand through a dreadfully painful and frightening ordeal. It was through these two simple forms of communication, in this intense situation, that I felt as though we had made some kind of connection. Although it sounds extremely overdramatic, in the immediate aftermath of that incident I recognised that there had been an almost spiritual connection. The need for him to know people's names suggests a need to know the people around him, to give him some security and comfort in his time of need.

Ronaldson (2000) describes moments such as these as times of spiritual searching and intensity which may occur in the hustle and bustle of everyday care. She states that nurses are involved in patients' spirituality every time we practice and our own spirituality is affected. Similarly, Eastbrooks and Morse (1992) state that the final phase of connection with a patient is touching, which they suggest is more than just the skin to skin contact. One informant actually described the completion of touching as "bumping souls". This is something similar to what I personally felt in the aftermath of the trauma. ...'

This moving reflective account helps us to understand the student's intense feelings in a traumatic situation and shows how she contributed to the care the young man received. She needed to explore the intensity of her emotions both verbally with her tutor and then further in a written form. She was able to make more sense of her experience by using a variety of perspectives and so this is an excellent example of how useful reflection can be. Her emotional and academic labour became an important resource in helping her to develop both personally and professionally.

The part identification may play in our emotional reactions.

In an earlier chapter, we described the sense of connection or identification we can have with particular patients and their families when we feel as if 'a button is pressed within us' and we feel especially linked to them. This can enable us to connect with them very quickly but can also uncover deep emotions within us. Some situations may be more significant and even problematic for us because they remind us of someone we love, perhaps someone who has died, and so we associate our feelings of loss with them. It may also make us more aware of our own mortality, for example, if they are of a similar age to us. The triggers for these emotions may be very unexpected as you will discover in the next incident written by Janice.

Case Study 4.5

'... the paramedics informed us that they were approaching the hospital with a patient who had undergone a cardiac arrest. Immediately my heart started to race as I had no previous experience of the situation and did not know what to expect. Initially I was excited and could not wait to witness such a new experience. The staff nurse and I made our way to the designated area and prepared for the arrival of the patient. At that time my main concern was that I would be asked to participate in the process and, to be honest, I did not give much thought to the fact that this was a person with a life and a family. When the patient arrived the staff nurse proceeded with basic life support and the doctor administered a drug. Approximately ten minutes of witnessing this, I thought about what I was seeing and silently congratulated myself on handling situation so well. Suddenly I stopped looking at the patient and looked at 'John'. He had the exact same pair of slippers on as my granddad wears. Well, that was it! I felt very sad and saw him as a person in his own right rather than just a patient who was receiving medical attention – I could easily have burst into tears right then and actively controlled the urge to get upset.'

Time to think back

+ How did Janice's emotions and thoughts change over the short period described?
+ What was the trigger which changed her feelings about John?
+ What was the benefit of the 'trigger' and what were the consequences of its impact on her?
+ What could have helped her cope with the situation?

It must have been very difficult for Janice to control her feelings, but given that she was involved in caring for a patient in a life-threatening situation as part of the team, she showed selflessness in controlling her feelings although we know that she found it helpful to talk about these intense feelings at a later time. All nurses may experience these unexpected triggers although they may be hidden from our awareness. We will go on to discuss these issues further.

Suzie, a newly qualified nurse, had a similar experience to Janice. Consider the following incident and jot down anything you think might have had an effect on her emotional state (consciously or unconsciously).

Case Study 4.6

'I was working on the accident and emergency department. I came on duty at 4 p.m. on Easter Sunday. I had spent the afternoon with my 4-year-old niece, opening Easter eggs and generally enjoying a great afternoon.

On arrival in the department I was confronted with the grieving parents of a 3-year-old girl, who had died by choking on a plastic toy from inside one of her eggs. I was told by the senior nurse to stay with the parents in the interview room and that they would want to see their child again. I felt very nervous because I had secretly avoided grieving relatives in the past and I now felt I did not have the special skills to deal with distressed relatives.

The parents were recently separated. The father of the child was aggressive and rather hysterical. Although I felt completely out of my depth and just did not know what to say, I stayed with them. The final stressor came when I accompanied the parents to see their daughter; she was wearing white socks with red hearts on them and they were the same as the ones my niece was wearing when I had left her an hour before.

Compare your considerations with ours

Suzie went from a happy scenario at home into a sad and distressing one at work. The closeness and immediacy of two contrasting environments which were connected by similarities (e.g. similar children, Easter eggs, and same patterned socks) made a particular impact. She was faced with the need to cope with grieving relatives – the father was described as 'aggressive' and 'hysterical'. She highlights the fact that she had avoided grieving relatives in the past. This may have been at an unconscious as well as a conscious level. Suzie recognised that the final trigger was the sock – a conscious reminder of the inevitability and unpredictability of death, even in her own family. She may have been unconsciously refusing to acknowledge this.

Suzie's experience was affected by the parallels she drew with her own family life and her difficulties in coping with issues related to death and dying. Her reactions and feelings of being out of her depth are common in such situations.

Long after it had happened to her, Salvage (2006: 26) described how she remembered with 'a shudder patients who I felt I had failed'. She had a mixture of feelings of anger and grief about a teenage girl who had suffered brain damage during a routine operation and later on was able to see that these feelings were tangled up with her grief for her brother who had died at the same age. She said: 'At the time I had no way of understanding this. We were offered no support or framework within which to express and explore the emotional and personal meanings of our work' (Salvage, 2006: 23). Because of this and of feeling undervalued, overworked and stressed, Salvage described how hard she felt it was to 'dig deep and find caring reserves', leading to what she described as 'compassion fatigue.'

Nowadays there are more opportunities for student nurses to discuss their feelings either with a mentor, tutor or other colleagues and sometimes through undertaking reflective exercises and assignments. However, the importance of these feelings can still be overlooked. If you see the relevance of this for your professional development, it will encourage you to make full use of a range of strategies, such as reflection, so that you are able to become more self-aware and turn your compassion into helpful nursing actions.

McCreight (2005) takes a positive view of this approach and confirmed the view that emotion should be seen as a resource rather than a weakness or deficit. She studied nurses and midwives who were helping women who had experienced miscarriage or stillbirth. She found they suffered grief and fear when dealing with the loss of a baby and some found it difficult to cope with the emotional distress. However, through analysing their personal feelings (she described this as emotional work), they were able to manage their emotions. She concluded that understanding the meaning of those emotions helped them to develop their professional understanding.

Graham *et al.* (2005) also described how a group of nurses were helped to uncover painful memories of caring for dying patients through reflection. They described the 'mutual suffering' nurses engaged in as a result of feelings of failure and the non-exposure of emotions. The sharing of these feelings through a reflective workshop helped them to conceptualise and articulate their nursing practice. 'The participants found that mutual suffering is a transformational process, leading to professional confusion and personal crisis but it also involves new beginings and clarification of values and beliefs' (Graham *et al.*, 2005: 283).

Time to think back

We have discussed the important part that emotions play in our practice and how emotional labour may be equally as demanding as physical labour:

+ Have you been underestimating the extent to which your emotions can both help and develop your understanding of practice?
+ Have you been using theoretical perspectives to help inform your practice and increase your awareness about emotional knowledge? In trying to make sense of a harrowing event, you may have noticed that the student who described her interactions with a young man who had been stabbed, used ideas from a variety of sources to help her to recognise and articulate her experience. You may also find it helpful to reflect on emotional 'triggers' in your own practice.
+ Have you found that certain sights, sounds or perhaps even smells have evoked in you an emotional response?
+ Reflecting on all this will help you to understand how important your emotions are in your practice.

Coping with difficult situations

As we have seen, we may find that caring for some people makes other kinds of emotional demands on us. It is natural to acknowledge feelings of anger, fear and even disgust at some of the things we may come across. As we saw in Chapter 3 in our discussion of anti-discriminatory practice, we have to be careful that we recognise these feelings and attitudes in ourselves so that we are able to 'manage' them and prevent them from interfering with the care we provide. The next story, told to us by Petra, a student nurse, illustrates this.

Case Study 4.7

'I was looking after Marge, a patient on an elderly mental infirm (EMI) unit. She was very difficult to nurse as she was extremely aggressive and abusive. It took a lot of time and patience to talk to her. Because of this I often felt that Marge was mainly left to be looked after by the students as the staff nurses did not have enough time.

One day I spent a great deal of time with her helping her to wash and dress. I sat for about twenty minutes persuading her to take her medication. Every half hour she was doubly incontinent and needed to be cleansed and changed. Her dressing gown was soiled and she didn't have another one. She started to shout at me to fetch her dressing gown for her. No matter how many times I pleasantly and firmly told her that the dressing gown she could see was not hers, but the lady's in the next bed, she continued to yell. She then shouted "You're a lazy bitch, I wish you would all f--- off and leave me."

I felt very annoyed and upset at this, but mainly disheartened because of all the time and effort I had put into giving her care even though I knew she couldn't really help it. ...'

Petra's story illustrates the mixture of emotions we might feel when we care for others. At one level she understood both Marge's predicament and her anger but she needed to feel her efforts were being recognised (the need for reciprocity as we discussed in Chapter 2). The story also illustrates that it is often demanding and complex care which is undertaken by the least experienced!

As we have said previously, an important part of our professional development is learning how to labour with and manage our emotions, and Petra is beginning to do that. This does not mean ignoring or rejecting her feelings but making an open and honest assessment of what they mean and how they might affect her practice. If we do not do this and are overcome by our emotions, we will feel let down when everything is not as perfect as we would like it to be and we will feel guilty about things we may not be able to do anything about. Conversely, by ignoring them we may disregard and dehumanise people and practise in a routine, unfeeling way in an effort to protect ourselves.

A study by Smith (2003) reveals that many students have some difficulty in disentangling what they see as 'personal emotions' from those expected of a 'professional' but see resolving this as an important part of their professional development. She cites a number of incidents that help demonstrate this, including the following episode written by a third year student.

'I had to act professionally in this situation because I don't know what I would have felt for this relative who was standing there looking all smart and smug when his wife was practically dying. (According to reports, she had been left for hours before an ambulance was called.) I think that if I hadn't been professional I think I would have said something wrong – I even felt like hitting him! I was so angry! That poor woman! Looking back on it, I think that it was so wrong of me to have felt that way. I don't think I should have felt so much anger towards him. We are taught not to be judgemental.'

To think about

You can see this third year student reflects back on her negative feelings and judgement about the patient's husband. She acknowledges she felt very angry with him and then guilty about these feelings, saying 'I think it was so wrong of me. ... We were taught not to be judgemental.'

✦ Have you been 'taught' not to be judgemental? What does this mean for you?
✦ How do you do this on a practical level, for example in a situation such as the above?
✦ Jot down your thoughts and compare them with ours.

Your reflections might be useful as part of your portfolio evidence, e.g. re. ethical dimensions.

As we discussed in Chapter 1, Smith (1992) described 'surface and deep acting' as part of emotional labour when there is a gap between what you do and what you may feel. This means that through emotional labour we can temporarily suspend our judgement of another's behaviour. By surface acting the student was labouring emotionally and acting at a 'surface level'. The student notes she was able to be professional and did not say anything 'wrong' to the husband – even though she 'even felt like hitting him' at one point.

This was positive in that she did not overtly express her feelings towards the husband of the patient, but as you are probably aware, non-verbal communication often 'leaks through' in our posture, eye contact and so on. She was able to temporarily suspend her judgemental attitude to some degree by this surface acting. We can also change the way we feel by re-arranging our thoughts. Labouring emotionally by 'deep acting' might have helped her, for example, when she felt anger and guilt. The student could have accepted that it is a normal everyday occurrence for us all to make judgements of value and worth about the world and the people in it – this comes from our own frame of reference, past experiences, influenced by our culture, peers, families, education and so on. She might then have acknowledged that she did not know the world of this relative. We therefore need to be very conscious of our feelings towards others and be aware of our prejudices and biases.

Rogers's (1961) description of 'unconditional positive regard' is helpful in this – it is an attitude of mind which makes us positive towards the people we work with, regardless of how we feel about them. Thompson (2002: 146) sums this up well. 'This does not mean that we have to like everyone we work with, or that we are 'not allowed' to have negative feelings, but it does mean that we need to be as effective as possible with all the people we work with, regardless of feelings towards them or what they may have done. Difficult though it may be to be positive towards people we do not like, good practice requires us to overcome these difficulties.' In other words, to be able act in a professional manner means that we have to be aware of and suspend our judgements, opinions and beliefs about how the world is. If we 'decentre' or move from our own world with its preoccupations and concerns we will be in a better position to assist those who require our help.

The importance of boundaries in care

Learning the boundaries of professional practice is also bound up with the emotions we feel for patients in our care. In our experience, students need a chance to explore situations in order to learn how professional boundaries can protect both patient and nurse.

An incident from a first year student nurse highlights this. The student had gone to meet a friend at the station when she saw a patient, who she knew was detained under the Mental Health Act and was particularly vulnerable, getting on a train. She was frightened about what might happen to the patient. Her first thoughts were to distance herself from the situation (she even thought about pretending she had not seen the patient trying to board the train) and yet she decided that, although off duty, she had to act in accordance with a caring, patient-oriented philosophy. She attempted to persuade the patient to go for a cup of coffee to gain time and when this was unsuccessful, she then thought about attempting to stop the train leaving by asking help from a member of the railway staff. She was trying to work within the professional NMC Code of Conduct concerning the need to protect the patient from harm but also thought about the need to maintain confidentiality. Eventually, a telephone call back to the hospital ward was effective in ensuring that strategies were put in place by the ward team and the patient returned safely to the hospital ward.

By talking through her fears and concerns at the time, the student was helped not only to consider the positive and the difficulties in her approach but also to consider professional expectations and boundaries. In nursing we engage in very close relationships some of which, by their very nature, move outside normal social conventions and barriers, for example in the kind of intimate care we give, or psychological support we provide based on confidential information or knowledge. We must always be sure that we act in the patient's interests and also protect ourselves from the likelihood of misunderstandings. As a student you need to be sure you read and understand any guidance given to staff in your area of practice. You will also find the NMC Code of Conduct (2008) a helpful guide. The student, in alerting the ward team to the possible dangers the patient was in, could be judged to have done what could reasonably be expected in this emergency situation.

Learning to keep your cool

Some of us, finding ourselves in a similar situation to the student at the railway station, may have distanced ourselves from the event. This is a form of detachment which may mean that we are actually holding back in order to protect ourselves. That may be a good thing in that we seem to have only a finite set of resources of energy upon which to draw. Part of our emotional labour may be concerned with maintaining a balance of being close, friendly, warm and approachable and maintaining professional distance. Being overfamiliar or too remote are both unacceptable. However, the detached position may not necessarily be a 'wrong place' to be, in that it may also, paradoxically, include a state of readiness for action.

As Goleman (1998) notes, those who have the ability to 'keep cool' are admired throughout the world. There are benefits to be gained from those who appear to 'stay collected' when there is an emergency, and/or there is distress or panic. Those who do this can bring a comforting sense of control to the situation. This is especially so if the situation requires immediate and concentrated actions, perhaps to save a life or reduce aggression. Being able to be objective in such situations is an essential part of professional development and also denotes a caring approach.

Sadly, sometimes nurses are on the receiving end of verbal abuse and physical violence. The NHS has recognised that the public should not expect health and social care workers to tolerate violence, bullying and aggression and the Department of Health launched a zero tolerance campaign tackling violence against staff in the NHS (Department of Health, 2002)

Beech and Leather (2003) note the importance of implementing and evaluating student nurse training related to this important aspect. The development of skills, debriefing and shared, supportive critical evaluation of responses and interventions will come some way in overcoming feelings of low morale and low self-esteem which may occur as a result of such occurrences. Nurses are ordinary people who, because of the challenging nature of their work, have to develop a range of coping skills in difficult situations and also antidotes to ameliorate negative behaviour arising from our distress. We have to learn to help each other to be objective, alter our mindset and work against our unhelpful responses so we can learn to educate our emotions and behaviours.

A certain 'state of readiness' is key if we are to demonstrate our willingness to deal with situations if and when they arise. Charlie wrote the next incident when she was a staff nurse new to a ward that specialised in vascular surgery. In fact Charlie told us that she was very cross with herself about what happened in this incident because her view of patient care 'has always been humanistic and we as nurses cannot afford to work on automatic pilot'. Read Charlie's story and before you read our explanation which follows, consider these points:-

+ Why did Charlie feel guilty and angry with herself?

+ What does the story tell us about 'being in a state of readiness'?

+ What does it tell us about the importance of non-verbal communication?

+ What prompted Bella's progression in the healing process?

Case Study 4.8

'I was working in the acute surgical area, on a late shift. In the afternoon the staffing levels were adequate as there was a reduced operating theatre list. This allowed more time than usual for patient care. The patient was one of fifteen on my team. Bella had had a left, above knee amputation due to peripheral vascular disease. The amputation was the second for Bella, who had needed the same surgery performed on her right leg two years previously. Bella was quite aware that this recent surgery was needed and stated prior to theatre that she was amazed that the second operation had not been performed at an earlier date. For a long time she had suffered from infected ulceration of her left leg and had experienced terrible pain. This had been poorly controlled by medication.

On this particular afternoon, the bandage on her wound site was to be reduced and observed by nursing staff. This was to check that the incision site was healing. As I reduced the bandages, I felt quite relaxed. Bella had experienced an amputation before; therefore I assumed that this would help her cope much better with the recent operation. However, unexpectedly, just as I was removing the tail end of the dressing, Bella burst into tears and started to wail. She declared herself to be an outcast and that she could not bear her present image. She held her hands over her face. My 'gut feeling' told me I needed to be close to Bella. I found myself 'entering her space' as I lowered my position so that our heights were equal. I met Bella at face level. I sat by her side so that she would know I had time and to be close enough for me to touch her hand as needed.

As we sat Bella's wails became gentle weeps. I felt the need to be even closer, so I moved my hand from my lap and held her hand. After this I took my hand from her hold and placed it gently on the site of her limb that had been recently removed.

Bella stopped crying immediately and there was a short silence. She looked at me initially with curiosity, perhaps shock, then said calmly in a loud voice, "I am still me aren't I, Charlie?"

Bella smiled and when she did this I smiled and said, "You will always be you Bella." After this incident occurred Bella slowly began to resume her usual behaviour. At further wound reviews she never again experienced such upset. She took positive interest in her physio-therapy and rehabilitation programme. I strongly believe that touching her leg after surgery, observing the wound incision and acknowledging the loss of her limb assisted her to come to terms with her altered body image.

Although I was pleased with Bella's progress, knowing that I had helped her, I felt torn and disturbed for days and weeks after the incident had occurred. How could I have assumed that this patient could cope better with that experience because it was not the first? She had lost her remaining leg! I felt frustrated at myself, I had honestly believed that Bella would 'know how' this surgery would affect her appearance. I now felt inconsiderate in my initial assump-tions. This has taught me that empathy is so very important.'

Compare your considerations with ours

Charlie felt angry with herself and guilty because she thought she ought to have anticipated that Bella would be distraught at losing her second limb through surgical amputation. Charlie detached herself from her focus on the task of wound dressing and recognised Bella's distress. Although taken by surprise, her state of readiness, due in part to her belief in the importance of humanistic care, meant that she was able and willing to disengage from being on 'automatic pilot' and respond to Bella effectively.

The importance of non-verbal communication and the sound and sight of Bella's clear distress signals prompted Charlie's action. She reacted by what she called 'entering into her space', moving her position so she was at the same level and close to Bella, by using touch (particularly of the affected limb) as a means of reassurance, acknowledgement and comfort.

The interaction between Bella and Charlie helped to progress the healing process. After the therapeutic touch, Bella's 'wails became gentle weeps' and she was suddenly able to step back from her emotions and remembered her own uniqueness. She asked the rhetorical question 'I am still me aren't I, Charlie?' She already knew the answer because Charlie had acknowledged her as a person. Her self-identity was re-established and this had a positive effect on the way she was able to engage in her physical rehabilitation. Nurses are engaged in work like this in all areas of nursing. They may be helping people who are suffering from altered self-image related to disfigurement from burns or other accidental injury, strokes, surgery or those with mental illness or learning disability.

You may be surprised in Charlie's story at how much effect a seemingly simple interaction can have. As we have found in earlier chapters, this kind of work is hidden and often undervalued even by ourselves. Considered analysis and critical reflection help us to uncover it. Through discussion and support, Charlie was able to see that being new to the ward had a bearing on her being unable to anticipate Bella's grief. The reflective process also helped her to become more self-aware and acknowledge the contribution she made to Bella's care. Otherwise she may have carried these guilt feelings around with her for a long period. She now better understands the need to be gentle with herself and learn from her emotions. She passes this message on to you:

> 'I hope that other nurses like me realise that it is acceptable to experience guilt, but to know that it also has a place. It is a major move forward for me within my clinical practice to identify and understand guilt more each day. Even though I remain quite critical of myself in clinical practice and find self-praise a difficult task, I hope in time that this will change. Since my experience of sharing and completing the reflective process I feel I have been able to combine personal and professionalism more than ever before. There are still more challenges to be completed in observing the 'self' further to improve my clinical practice. The more nurses experience these situations, the more they can identify with the uniqueness of patients such as Bella, but without forgetting their own being.'

Linking theory and practice

We can see how reflection helps us to uncover important and valuable aspects of nursing. Some might say it teaches us about what care is really all about. It helps us to identify the range of caring skills which help people like Bella and influence their progress. You may have thought of a variety of perspectives which would help shed light on Charlie and Bella's story such as theories and information about empathy, body image, self-identity and its influence on rehabilitation, non-verbal communication and preparation for surgery. Theories and the evidence base for practice can be wide-ranging and varied – this is what makes nursing so interesting and complex. We thought it might also be useful to carry the discussion a little further.

A significant moment in the story occurred when Bella observed herself and wondered if she was still the same person as she was before the second amputation. Charlie also asked herself questions about her own ability and this led to feelings of anger and guilt which would have affected her self-esteem and therefore self-image. A positive outcome was that she eventually saw her emotional world as a useful focus for learning about herself. Griffin and Tyrrell (2003) claim that we all have an 'observing self' and this is probably the most significant difference between human beings and the rest of the animal kingdom. They suggest that nature has supplied us with this as a therapeutic restorative – just as both Bella and Charlie found. Discussing the application of their view to therapeutic work, they suggest that, 'This is because the observing self is a more fundamental part of us than even our thinking and feeling selves. It is our awareness that everything else feeds into. A person can lose arms, legs, sight, hearing and yet still have that sense of 'I am', and being a centre of experience of reality – 'I am aware'. ... All good therapists have the skill to help the client step back into their observing self (even if they don't call it by that name) to identify patterns of conditioning that need to change' (Griffin and Tyrrell, 2003: 87).

The story of Charlie and Bella helps show us that if we have warmth, regard, certain understandings and skills we can help to disengage others and ourselves from emotional, dazed-like states. Our observing self can help us gain a more objective/neutral/unbiased view of our world. This state or way of being is potentially therapeutic as a conscious, logical mind can better objectively check out feelings. In this frame of mind it is possible to question, to scrutinise the situation at hand and to solve problems in more creative ways. In summary, this will help us visualise and plan ways of providing better care.

Another perspective that we might use to help our understanding is that of Goleman (1998: 136-137) who comments that when we start to connect or communicate with each other we begin 'to fall into a subtle dance of rhythmic harmony'. Movements, postures, vocal pitch, rate of speaking, and even the length of pauses between one person speaking and the other's response become synchronised. Indeed, in the latter part of the incident, we see Bella taking some control over this synchronisation process. It is as if Bella returns Charlie's understanding and compassionate care by smiling at her, a tribute or thank you to Charlie, and Charlie smiled back – 'in a subtle dance of harmony'. As Goleman (1998: 167) asserts, 'Smiling is the most contagious emotional signal of all, having an almost irresistible power to make other people smile in return.'

The work of Rogers (1961) also helps us better understand the abilities and skills associated with empathy. These competencies are about being able to enter the client's world and help them and also being able to get out of the situation without being scathed – that is without being injured or traumatised. Reflection can help us to do this. On a similar note, Goleman (1998: 317) argues that we have emotional intelligence which includes 'the ability to recognise our own feelings as well as those of others, for motivating ourselves, and for managing emotions well in ourselves and in our relationships'. If we are to work together effectively as a team, we also have a responsibility to colleagues in helping them to cope with emotional situations.

Helping colleagues to cope

As a student, you probably get a great deal of help from other students who share similar fears and concerns to yours. A third year student told us how she observed a way in which some qualified staff helped each other.

Case Study 4.9

'I was thinking the other day about the ways we survive in nursing and saw more clearly that detaching from all of the emotional baggage is not all that bad. I thought about some of the theories I knew from the literature, such is Pam Smith's research on the emotional labour of nursing and also the 'hot action', as Eraut describes aspects of our work when we are so busy we can hardly think straight. I reflected on my own beliefs that we have to learn to detach as a way of protecting ourselves; otherwise we can find ourselves in some sort of 'burnout' position.

I started to see that nurses do 'detach' themselves in various ways from it all, otherwise it gets too much. I know that we need to be careful about doing this, because it is so easy to start seeing patients and relatives as less than people and that can be so dangerous. On the other hand, we do need to look after ourselves and I think that this might be an almost 'unseen feature' of our work.

For example, on our ward recently Wendy, the staff nurse, said to the ward sister, 'If you don't mind, I won't go into that cubicle today as I have got a bit of a cold.' The sister agreed with Wendy straight away, saying it was fine and that Wendy looked a 'bit under the weather today'. I honestly do not think that Wendy had a cold. She had been caring for a baby who had died the previous day and wanted to keep her distance from any more emotional stuff, until she felt strong again and ready to face a new challenge.

I believe that the ward sister knew this was the reason Wendy did not want to go into the cubicle. And Wendy knew that this sister saw past the 'I have a cold' excuse. But the cold excuse is a shorthand way of saying 'I need to be protected'.'

As students, you may find there are several people who help a great deal in giving you support in your 'emotional labour'. As well as peers, perhaps you have gained help from a really good mentor, or a personal tutor. Smith and Gray (2001: 233) undertook a study of student nurses and found that link tutors (who visited the students in practice) were helpful. They did this not only by liaising with senior clinical staff and mentors on behalf of the students but also in encouraging reflective learning and informal support, often by identifying with student experiences. 'If my student is having a hard time with a really ill patient, it helps if I can link that with the difficulties I have had. That way you feel you actually feel more about it and can relate to the student. It helps to work it through with them and see what to do next.'

Just as we've been able to learn a great deal from nurses' stories throughout this book so, it would seem, the very act of telling the story helps to clarify significant events. It is also interesting that Smith and Gray found that students and mentors found it easier to talk about good practice than to write about it. Perhaps it is the informality of sharing stories and ideas that makes this a particularly useful strategy and allows us to uncover details we might otherwise have overlooked. The authors concluded that the role of reflection, storytelling and the use of oral accounts are ways of accumulating evidence to demonstrate the content and process of emotional labour in teaching, learning and caring. Mentors and link tutors have a central role in ensuring this occurs. However, this is a two-way process. As a student, how you react to your mentor, tutors and other colleagues, will influence your learning experience by, for example, whether you are able and willing to engage in reflective conversations. In later chapters, we will be discussing more about how you might develop your ability to do this by finding ways of increasing your self-awareness and becoming more analytical about your emotional reactions to situations.

Summary

In this chapter, we have explored the emotional world of nursing and have seen the relevance of acknowledging and using our emotions as a resource for developing our caring skills.

+ We have found that the emotional world of nursing can be demanding but also intensely satisfying.

+ We have seen how nurses, engaged in everyday tasks which bring them close to patients, can help overcome problems related to self-image.

+ We have learned more about the part emotions can play in the way in which nurses see their practice and react to situations, including the way they make judgements and behave.

+ Identification with particular patients and objects can act as triggers and affect our emotional balance.

+ We have seen the importance of using opportunities for reflective learning both for ourselves and for others. This includes gaining more understanding of parameters of our professional relationship with service users and their families.

Looking forward

A major focus of care in all branches of nursing is related to people with long-term health care needs. Because of this, most of this care now takes place in the community and is likely to increase even further in the future. In the next chapter, we will explore the challenges of developing caring and effective relationships with service users and their carers. These are people with vast experience and we need to capture and utilise this. More care is undertaken by informal carers, perhaps assisted by multi-professional teams, and so care in the community is an important aspect of your experience as a student – in some branches of nursing a predominant feature. We will use stories from service users, students and qualified nursing staff to help us learn more about the way in which we can develop effective and supportive caring partnerships by pooling our knowledge and resources.

Activity

Look at the caring indicators and use them to explore your own emotional world of practice. You may find them useful to prompt your reflections, either verbally or in a written form. The aim of this activity will be for you to see how knowledge of your emotions will help you to improve your caring skills.

Caring indicators

1. Willingness to use your emotional labour as a resource for developing caring skills – ability to turn compassion into effective nursing actions

2. Being in a state of readiness for action

3. 'Keeping cool' in stressful situations

4. Recognising 'triggers' in specific events

5. Providing effective reassurance, support and comfort in a variety of ways, e.g. through appropriate touch and verbal communication

6. Assisting in the 'dance of rhythmic harmony' by mirroring the other, e.g. by smiling, synchronising postures, movements, vocal pitch and rate of speaking and length of pauses

7. Finding ways of coping with or managing upsetting situations

8. Using opportunities to promote a patient's positive self-image

9. Maintaining a balance of emotions, being neither hardened nor overemotional

10. Keeping within the boundaries of professional practice

11. Helping colleagues with emotional labour, e.g. by passing on tacit or hidden practice knowledge which adds to our caring skills

---

References

Beech, B and Leather, P (2003) Evaluating a management of aggression unit for student nurses. *Journal of Advanced Nursing* **44**, 603-612.

Department of Health (2007) NHS zero tolerance campaign tackling violence against staff in the NHS. DoH.

Eastbrooks, C and Morse, J (1992) Toward a theory of touch: the touching process and acquiring a touching style, *Journal of Advanced Nursing* **17**, 448-456

Gibson, M and Iwaniec, D (2003) An empirical study into the psychosocial reactions of staff working as helpers to those affected by the aftermath of two traumatic incidents. *British Journal of Social Work* [online] **33**, 851-870. Available from www.proquest.umi.com (accessed 3 July 2007).

Goleman, D (1998) *Working with Emotional Intelligence*. London: Bloomsbury.

Graham, I, Andrewes, T and Clark, L (2005) Mutual suffering: a nurse's story of caring for the living as they are dying. *International Journal of Nursing Practice* **11**, 277-285.

Griffin, J and Tyrrell, I (2003) *Human Givens: A new approach to emotional health and clear thinking*. Chalvington, UK: HG Publishing.

James, N (1992) Care = organisation + physical labour + emotional labour. *Sociology of Health and Illness* **14**, 488-505.

McCreight, B (2005) Perinatal grief and emotional labour: a study of nurses' experience in gynae wards. *International Journal of Nursing Studies* **42**, 439-448.

NMC (Nursing and Midwifery Council) (2008) *The Code: Standards of conduct, performance and ethics for nurses and midwives.* London: NMC.

Parkinson, F (1997) *Critical Incident Debriefing: Understanding and dealing with trauma.* London: Sovenir Press.

Phillips, S (1996) Labouring the emotions. *Journal of Advanced Nursing* **24**, 139-143.

Rogers, C (1961) *On Becoming a Person.* London: Constable.

Ronaldson, S (2000) *Spirituality: The Heart of nursing.* Parkville, Vic.: Ausmed Publications.

Salvage, J (2006) It's the action that counts. *Nursing Standard* **20**, 20-23.

Schutz, S, Angove, C and Sharp, P (2004) Assessing and evaluating reflection. In Bulman, C and Schutz, S (eds) *Reflective Practice in Nursing.* Oxford: Blackwell.

Smith, A (2003) Learning about reflection. PhD thesis. Northumbria University, Newcastle upon Tyne.

Smith, A and Russell, J (1991) Using critical incidents in nurse education. *Nurse Education Today* **11**, 284-291.

Smith, P (1992) *The Emotional Labour of Nursing: How nurses care.* London: Macmillan.

Smith, P and Gray, B (2001) Reassessing the concept of emotional labour in student nurse education: the role of link lecturers and mentors in a time of change. *Nurse Education Today* **21**, 230-237.

Strauss, A, Fagerhaugh, S, Suczek, B and Weiner, C (1982) Sentimental work in the technologised hospital. *Sociology of Health and Illness* **4**, 254-277.

Thompson, N (2002) *People Skills.* Basingstoke: Palgrave Macmillan.

Chapter 5

Creating caring partnerships with service users and their families

LEARNING OBJECTIVES

By the end of this chapter you should have an understanding of:

1. Creating effective partnerships with carers and those receiving care
2. The challenges of, and opportunities for, sustaining caring approaches within changing political, economic and social contexts
3. The importance of having a blend of caring attitudes, knowledge and competent skills in caring for others
4. How multi-professional and multi-agency approaches effect experiences of caring
5. Ways in which theory can help us to guide and reflect critically on practice

Introduction

It is easy to forget just how much care is undertaken by informal carers - partners, parents, daughters, sons, friends and neighbours who do so out of love and perhaps a sense of duty. The 2001 Census (Department of Health, 2005) gives us some understanding of this, indicating that there are approximately 5.2 million people in the UK who provide unpaid care for a relative, friend or neighbour and, in doing so, make a significant contribution to the care provided in the community. The largest group of carers are in the fifties age range, and over a million of these spend 50 hours a week or more on providing care. The increase in the number of people requiring help is related to greater life expectancy and medical success in treating people, including children, with chronic illnesses. There has also been a decrease in the number of hospitals and institutions for people with long-term needs. It is therefore important that, as professional carers, we are able work with and support informal carers effectively. In this chapter we will consider how nurses can help to sustain caring approaches, taking into account changes to their workplace and role from hospital to community, from providing direct care to helping and supporting others who give it for most of the time. We will explore the nature of the relationship between professionals, service users and informal carers, and consider the opportunities for, and challenges of, creating effective partnerships. Stories based on experience will continue to help us understand better ways of helping people and how we can use resources and theoretical frameworks to ensure we are caring in our approaches.

Living with a member of the family who has dementia

Caring for a relative with dementia may bring with it many emotional, physical, economic and social demands, which can occur over a prolonged period of time. With increased longevity has come a rise in the number of people suffering from Alzheimer's disease and so often the main carer may be older partners, with health problems themselves. Feelings such as guilt, frustration, concern, loss of hope and a sense of helplessness may arise for the carer as well as for the person suffering from dementia who may also experience loss of self-identity and self-esteem. This is more likely if the carer is under a great deal of stress and is unable to cope with situations which may arise.

Consider the following account written by a student nurse and think about the main issues which need to be considered. Compare your responses with ours.

Case Study 5.1

'We were asked to visit Harriet who had been discharged from hospital following a chest infection but had also been diagnosed with Alzheimer's disease. She lived with her daughter Rosie and her family. Rosie met us at the door and was close to tears. "I feel I'm at the end of my tether," she said. "I've been up half the night. At 3 a.m. I heard Mum – she had turned the radio on full blast and was sweeping the stairs. I tried to reason with her – and told her that it was the middle of the night – she became very stubborn – told me that it was the morning and she had to make an early start and get the work done. Eventually I persuaded her to sit down and have a cup of tea and then managed to get her back to bed but I couldn't get to sleep myself as I was worried that she would get up and turn the gas cooker on as she did a night or so ago. She seems much worse since she has been ill with the chest infection. My sister comes in to help as I go out to work and we really wanted to be able to look after her ourselves but we're finding it very difficult to cope!"'

Compare your considerations with ours

More and more people find themselves in this situation, particularly women who are in full or part-time employment but try to do a 'juggling act' by also looking after relatives who need care. Rosie needs help if she is to continue to be able to care for her mother. The immediate need is to respond empathetically to her distress and talk through strategies to get practical help.

You may have wondered what Harriet thought about all this and the level at which she might be functioning or be helped to function. Despite any cognitive impairment she might have, it is important to remember that a sense of self can be retained even at the very end stages of dementia. This has been described by Kitwood (1997) as a sense of personhood which is underpinned by feelings of personal worth, a sense of agency (which means that he or she can still make things happen), social confidence and acceptability, and hope. She should be given an opportunity to participate in decisions and arrangements made about her care if she is able. Aggarwal et al. (2003: 188) highlight ways which will help us to access views and feelings of those with dementia, including 'adapting to their pace and timescale, taking account of environmental factors and studying non-verbal communication'. This will help not only Harriet but also Rosie and the rest of the family.

You may also have questioned the quality of the discharge planning. There may have been pressure on bed occupancy within the hospital so Harriet may have been discharged as soon as her acute medical condition (chest infection) improved with very little thought or planning into how the condition and hospitalisation might have had an impact on her overall level of functioning. More communication between the hospital and community team might have helped and a full assessment of her functioning and well-being, perhaps by using a tool such as dementia care mapping (Kitwood and Bredin, 1992).

You might also have considered the blurring of the boundaries between health and social care. Who will take responsibility to help Harriet and Rosie? Multi-agency work is a key factor here and consideration has to be given to determine which professional colleagues and agencies will be able to help best in assessing, planning and implementing a care package. A social work referral is essential if this has not yet occurred. Caring in this case might be helping Rosie to explore the resources available to her. There are numerous websites which are useful for this including the Department of Health website on www.direct.gov.uk, or carers' websites such as www.carersuk.org or www.dementialink.org which will give Rosie (and you) information on carers' rights, financial support and national and local support groups.

Linking theory and practice

As Rosie feels she is at 'the end of her tether' she needs as much help as possible if she is to be able to continue to care for her mother. Marion Witton (2003), a nurse herself, provided a moving account of her own family's experiences of coping with her mother who was diagnosed as suffering from Alzheimer's disease. She suggests that there is time when a family is able to recognise this. She described the effect on the family of many distressing changes in her mother who became depressed and anxious, lost her memory, complained a lot, became self-absorbed, having no interest in anyone but herself, and dependent on her husband, not letting him out of her sight. Marion wrote: 'It is never easy to have to accept 'outside' help in the form of services. The emotions of dealing with the deterioration of a loved one and the feeling of 'failure' to do everything yourself are hard to admit' (2003: 15). A caring nurse will recognise this and, working in partnership with families and as a member of a supportive team, will help a family to cope. In Marion's case, her family was helped to turn a distressing situation into a manageable one. She explained this as follows. 'Nothing was imposed. The many people involved through the health care and the voluntary sectors were efficient yet understanding and caring. The legislation and ethos of community care worked for us in that what was given was not just to the patient but to the whole family' (2003: 15).

Marion's experience reflects positive work which is taking place to support families in caring ways. As mentioned in earlier chapters, a significant amount of care, particularly within the community, is still provided by women, although, with the changing role of women in society with more engaged in full time work and also interested in career advancement, the balance may be changing (Morrison and Bennett, 2006). Nevertheless, there is still an expectation that a woman will take on reponsibility for the caring role and this usually falls to a daughter although if a son is the nearest or only next of kin, it may well be a daughter-in-law. The expectation of caring as 'women's work' may account for it being seen as 'natural', 'their duty' and 'unskilled'. As we have seen, however, it may not be an easy or a short-term task. Taking responsibility for the care of another person, of whatever age group, may last a number of years and may be very challenging. In addition, many middle-aged women may now not only find themselves responsible for the care of an older relative but also caring for preschool grandchildren. Professionals, therefore, have to work closely with carers and draw on multi-professional and voluntary resources if they are to support families within the community and help maintain the quality of life for carers as well as those being cared for.

There may be other difficulties in that if family members caring for an older person continue working, they may find that their employer's 'family friendly' policies and practices are not designed to address the needs of staff members who care for older and disabled adults as they are more likely to be geared towards the needs of working parents of young children, although even this may be difficult.

To think about

+ Who does the caring in your family?
+ What does this entail?
+ What are the implications in terms of possible stresses but also the benefits?

You may have found that, in your family, caring is shared amongst members of the family and although more men are now taking on a caring role, many women continue to take a major role in this even if they are in paid employment. Caring for someone usually involves a mixture of physical, emotional and social tasks. You may have highlighted tasks such as personal help with washing, shopping, cleaning, cooking or providing meals, paying bills, taking someone out, keeping them company, comforting and ensuring they are safe and protected. This is a way of demonstrating love or regard for a person, or could be undertaken out of a sense of duty. Rewards from care-giving include seeing others benefiting from the care we provide and helping to create an environment where others can develop and/or cope with difficult situations. Carers may then feel positive about themselves as they are developing or continuing satisfying relationships. This is all part of the process of giving and receiving in care, as discussed in Chapter 2.

Caring can be hard work, and requires complex and wide-ranging skills. It can be emotionally very demanding, restrict social opportunities for carers and cause stress and worry. Phillips *et al.* (2002) studied the impact on women working as formal carers (in health and social care) but who also had responsibilities as informal carers (suggesting perhaps that being a nurse or a social worker might mean that other members of the family delegate the responsibility of care to them). These authors found that the majority of the women did not allow their caring responsibilities to have an impact on their work which sometimes acted as a buffer and was important for the women carers in terms of self-esteem and identity. However, the increasing demands on them were more likely to affect their family life and their own health, particularly in terms of stress and tiredness.

Support on the practical and emotional level, including supportive friends, colleagues and managers (who helped keep things in perspective), assisted them in being able to juggle the responsibilities of many competing demands but they also needed key organisational skills, e.g. in making out rotas. Phillips *et al.* found that seemingly straightforward strategies helped the women to cope and to 'avoid care overload'. Such strategies included being able to talk over problems with someone else, being able to draw not only on their own expertise but also on the experience they were building up, seeing the funny side of a situation and maintaining their outside interests. This study has important lessons for us in terms of what we may be called upon to do in both our personal and our professional lives and what is helpful to enable carers to continue to care in the community. As men take on more of such responsibilities, we also need to recognise that needs, particularly those of older men giving care, are complex and may be gender-specific (Witucki-Brown *et al.* 2007). They may, for example, be reluctant to ask for help or have feelings of inadequacy if they do so.

In Chapter 2 we described the study by Brouwer *et al.* (2005) who found that, instead of seeing it as a burden, many informal care-givers reported positive benefits from providing care to their loved one and that on average their happiness levels would decline if this care was handed over to someone else. It is in the interest of everyone, therefore, to work effectively in partnership with carers such as Rosie to help maintain the positive benefits of providing care.

Creating caring partnerships with carers

As professionals we must ensure that we work with families as equal partners. If professionals disregard what may be seen as something as straightforward and basic as conventional good manners, the partnership will seem one-sided and disrespectful. You can see evidence of this in Gudrun's story.

Case Study 5.2

'We were due to have a meeting at the family home with a social worker and the specialist health visitor; an educational officer was also invited to attend.

Firstly, the health visitor could not remember what time the meeting was to be held so she called at ten minutes past eight in the morning. My husband let her in and she told him "I am just going to wait until the meeting starts". The meeting was actually at 9.30 a.m. So, basically she sat in the middle of our living room. It was the usual total morning chaos in our house (with people running around half dressed and trying to get the others out to school and work).

The problem for me was that she seemed to have disregarded the fact that we were a family and she was treating us as a 'case'. The fact that this was in our home seemed to be totally irrelevant to her and she did not value our privacy and show us respect.

We are not a 'disabled project' or a 'disabled family'; we are a family who happens to have a disabled child.'

You can see the way Gudrun has used particular language to describe the differences between how she views her situation and how she thinks the health visitor viewed her family. Simply by not arriving at a more appropriate time or even apologising, Gudrun feels that the needs and privacy of her family have not been appreciated and respected. Gudrun also thought her problems would be helped if professionals worked together as a team, sharing information and assessing the whole family's needs.

Case Study 5.3

'We want a joined up approach to our care; I get sick of repeating the same information to all of the professionals who visit us. There should be one person who can take the information and share it. I know they need profession-specific details, but there is a central core of information that they all want! For example, Billy has a physiotherapist, an occupational therapist, a paediatrician, a speech therapist, a dietician, a peripatetic educationalist for the visually impaired and receives 'formal care' during the day when I am at work (this carer has a qualification in nursery nursing and has looked after Billy since he was two).

I think this is important for student nurses to consider in that, once qualified, they may play a central role in the assessment and organisation of care needs for the child and family. The nurse really can 'get it all together' for the family; if they do their job properly. For us this would include information about how Billy's younger sister is affected by this. All of her life it has been "hang on till we do this for Billy and that for Billy". Sometimes it feels like it is me against the system and it should not be like that; the nurse would help me with the advocacy required to get what Billy needs. This is what I think the government means by a joined up approach. This is not what happens now, irrespective of what and how professionals are taught at the moment.'

It appears that the government has recognised the importance of supporting informal carers like Gudrun and is listening to what they are saying.

Time to think back

+ Jot down and/or search out government policies which are aimed at helping carers and ensure that they receive a 'joined-up' approach to care. Compare your findings with ours.
+ See how this might be applicable to your practice areas and how this information might be helpful as part of your evidence base for your ongoing assessment record/practice portfolio and help you to achieve the NMC proficiencies.

These are some of the policies we thought would be useful (you may have found more):

+ The Carers (Equal Opportunties) Act 2004 identified that the needs of carers should be taken fully into account in the assessment process.
+ This was followed by a White Paper *Our Health, Our Care, Our Say* (DoH, 2006) in which the Department of Health conducted an extensive public consultation which revealed considerable support for more recognition of the support needed for carers.
+ This led to the *New Deal for Carers* (DoH, 2007) which funded projects aimed at improving support for carers through a range of measures including establishing a helpline to offer advice to carers and proposing that short-term, home-based breaks to support carers in crisis or emergency situations were established in each council area.

✦ Specific funding for the creation of an expert carer's programme was also allocated. The rationale given for this was that caring is a role that is often taken on suddenly, leaving carers to struggle with the vital responsibilities that they have assumed without preparation. The aim of the *Expert Carer's Programme* (ECP) is to provide vital training to carers and will be available both by face-to-face and by distance learning, empowering carers by informing them of their rights, services available to them, developing their advocacy skills and their ability to network with other carers to support their needs.

As the nature of care work changes, the skills needed to help others fulfil a caring role change too. If followed through effectively, government policies can be extremely helpful in supporting and guiding carers, but as we know, many people need help to avail themselves of the opportunities present and may still need one-to-one advice from a health or social care professional. Nurses are in an excellent position to provide this.

As nurses, we are aware that there may be other considerations to take into account as increasingly, with demographic changes in society and an ageing population, sometimes the 'carer' may also be a person who is receiving 'care' themselves or, conversely, the care-provider may be a child.

Children as carers

Read Sharon and Roberto's story summarised below and consider what effect you think caring for his mother might have on Roberto in terms of his development and quality of life. Then compare your considerations with ours.

Case Study 5.4

Roberto is 10 years old and lives with his mother, Sharon, who suffers from a bipolar affective disorder. Sharon's illness means that at times she can be overactive and emotionally very 'high' and at other times she is very depressed and finds it difficult to be motivated to do anything, even to get up in the morning. She is embarrassed about her illness and because she feels friends and neighbours would not understand it, and would probably think she is 'not right in the head', she tends to keep herself to herself and socialise very little. There are no other members of the family living close by. Although the medication helps to control her mood swings, she is sometimes unable to undertake the usual activities of living such as cooking, shopping, cleaning etc., and this then falls to Roberto. Sharon feels guilty about her reliance on Roberto and told us, 'I've tried my best but I know I ask him to do too much. I try and make sure he is still able to enjoy himself but if I need help, he is the one who I rely on. He does all sorts of things – he can cook a meal, make a cup of tea, do the shopping and clean up. He cheers me up and makes me laugh when I'm down. He gets me to do things I wouldn't otherwise feel like doing – like taking my medication.' Sharon says she is a little wary of professionals. When she has been hospitalised in the past, Roberto received respite care and she is very frightened that he might be taken into care permanently.

Mick is a community psychiatric nurse who became Sharon's key worker. He recognised the close relationship between mother and son and made a point of spending time talking with Roberto to see what he thought about the situation and assess the effect it was having on him. Roberto felt that Mick was looking after both of them.

'He told me I was doing a good job with Mum and told me anything I needed to know about what was happening to her and what I should do in an emergency or if I was worried about anything. Sometimes I get a bit miffed if I can't get out to football practice when Mum needs me at home but most of the time it's OK – we sort things out. Mick got Annie, the social worker to come and see me and she got me to join the young carers support group at Barnardo's. It's good to talk to other kids in the same boat and we have a laugh!'

Compare your considerations with ours

You may have been concerned about Roberto, wondering about the effects that having so much responsibility might have on his psychological, social and educational development. You may think that he is 'losing his childhood' and the opportunities to enjoy himself with his peers. However, you will have also noticed that Roberto sees positive as well as negative effects. This was helped by having positive feedback from Mick so he feels recognised and appreciated for his efforts. Mick gave Roberto information which helped him to look after his mother better. This is an indication of an equitable and non-patronising partnership.

You might also have considered Sharon's role as a caring mother. The relationship between mother and son is one of closeness and it is therefore one of giving and receiving for both partners – one of mutuality and reciprocity as we saw in Chapter 2. Roberto is still receiving love and interest from his mother, although at times this might be hard to show in a physical sense, looking after the whole family means that Sharon is more likely to able to fulfil her role as a mother.

Mick worked effectively with Annie the social worker so that, through joining a young carer's group, there was an opportunity for Roberto to feel he had something in common with other children and could gain support and social benefits.

Using research to gain more knowledge

More knowledge about possible effects on Roberto and Sharon can be gained from Aldridge and Becker (2003) who conducted a study of children and young people under 18 years old who were caring for parents with enduring mental health problems. They came up with some interesting findings. A prime concern of the parents in the study related to the prognosis of their illness and how this would affect their children. They were concerned that the children lacked support when they were undertaking care and the authors considered that this could become an enduring and stressful aspect of the parents' mental ill health experience and could in turn create further crises for the family. Aldridge and Becker found, however, that whilst mental illness may result in loss of parenting function or that a child has to fulfil parent-like roles, as seems apparent with Sharon and Roberto, it can also cement parent–child relationships. They suggest that there is a need to improve our understanding of children's experience of caring when parents are affected by illness as these relationships are often perceived by professionals in health and social care as negative.

Consulting children themselves can uncover positive as well as adverse experiences, e.g. that providing the care themselves reduces some of their anxieties and fears. 'Our evidence shows that the damaging effects of children caring for and living with parents with mental health problems are not determined by the mental illness in itself and of itself, but by a range of other factors including isolation and exclusion (from care plans, service interventions, approaches from family and professionals and community misunderstanding and discrimination in particular), as well as by other social determinants (including low income, poverty and so on' (Aldridge and Becker 2003: 95). Children, they claim, may suffer from information deficit (and information should be provided in a way which is age-related) and that 'whole family' approaches should be used so that they are both consulted and can talk to someone whom they can trust and whom understands their needs both as children and as carers. There is evidence from their research that professionals across a range of disciplines felt able and competent to describe the effects on children based on their assumptions and not through close contact with children and their families. Therefore, although there is acknowledgement that some effects on children may be detrimental, there is call for professionals to use effective assessment and intervention strategies which will give children some degree of choice in undertaking care responsibilities. Roberto's story reinforces the need for us not to make assumptions about who is able or not able to provide care and to recognise the complexities and variety of care relationships.

Time to think back

+ Caring as taking account of whole family needs.
+ Respecting the privacy of the family and their right to make decisions about their care.
+ Not making assumptions but listening to what people say.
+ Being aware of resources which may help.
+ Communicating and working effectively with other professionals for the good of the family.

The complexity of caring partnerships

For some families who are struggling to care, there may be many difficulties which complicate the relationship between them and the professionals who try to help them. Susan, a student in placement with the community children's nursing team, told us about problems that arose when working with Ami and her family. Read her story, make a note of the difficulties and then compare your thoughts with ours.

Case Study 5.5

'Ami was born prematurely to Stephanie and Liam, who are a very young mother and father, both still in their teens. Before she had Ami, Stephanie had been 'sleeping rough' on the streets and it is believed she probably had taken drugs on a regular basis before and during part of her pregnancy. My mentor said that because Ami had been born early and had cerebral palsy and epilepsy she was kept in the special care baby unit and had to be fed via a nasogastric tube. Stephanie and Liam only stayed for a short time when they visited Ami and the social worker assisted the nurses in arranging a meeting with them to encourage them to get involved with feeding Ami via the tube so she could go home with them. This proved easier said than done as the parents sometimes failed to attend the unit for the teaching sessions and, when they did, it seemed to be a very difficult 'task' for them, in part due to Ami's very jerky thrashing arm movements and poor head control. Because of these problems the community children's team was involved prior to and after Ami's discharge from hospital.

When we visited Ami at home we found that both parents were insistent that they were managing very well 'thank you' and adamant that they gave her tube feeds according to the dietician's plan, although my mentor was concerned because Ami was not putting on weight. Stephanie in particular seemed to be not worried about this, appeared disinterested and did not seem to have bonded with Ami. She got very angry when my mentor asked questions, such as, were they having any problems feeding Ami during the night and would they like for the dietician to review the feeding regime? I thought to myself that it must be a difficult task because Ami had a lot of very strong thrashing arm movements and head movements so the tube often came out. Also, I reflected that because both parents were teenagers they might find it difficult to get up during the night for feeds. During another visit we noticed redness on the back of Ami's head and it became apparent that the reason for these was that she was laid on the floor for long periods. Stephanie and Liam took a long time convincing that the redness was caused because her head was thrashing around and rubbing against the hard floor matting. I saw for myself how difficult it was for the nurses to promote a trusting partnership type of relationship with Stephanie and Liam. They had to be so careful how, when and why they gave advice and/or intervened but they also had to be very aware of child protection issues.

Difficulties for Ami and her family

We thought the following difficulties should be taken into account (you may have come up with more).

+ Ami is a premature baby with complex health needs.

+ Ami was in hospital for some time and separated from her parents – attachment and bonding will have been affected.

+ Possibility of a child at risk.

+ The sparse visiting by Stephanie and Liam may be an indication that they are frightened of having a sick baby and being responsible for her care or may be related to the loss (absence) of a healthy child.

+ Tube feeding reinforced that the child was sick and different and required high level practical skills to care for her.

+ Stephanie had been sleeping rough during pregnancy suggesting that she may have very little social support and may still be in need of help to provide a stable, consistent environment.

The challenges for the nurses therefore included:

+ Need for effective risk assessment and to use knowledge about child protection issues and strategies, based on effective multidisciplinary working.

+ Problems in communication with parents in forming a relationship built on trust which is supportive and one in which parenting skills can be taught/learned and monitored.

+ Consideration of what strengths, resources and solutions would be useful.

Caring for Ami therefore involves taking into account so many aspects. We know that some families are resilient and more capable than others in coping with extreme stress and adversity. However, any family, faced with the situation of Stephanie and Liam would need help to build up their family strengths and resouces. You will find many studies related to family resilience in sociological and psychological literature. Patterson (2002) considers families as a 'social system' built upon a network of interrelationships, values and beliefs. Belonging to a family is a source of physical and psychological nurture and Ami needs to grow up in a family where, amongst other important things, she is loved and kept safe. Communication with Stephanie and Liam, and between all professionals involved in their care, is of vital importance if the family is to be helped to function well. This will include an accurate assessment of their capabilities and of the ways in which they view the situation. Recognising successes, however small, is crucial (Patterson, 2002).

Patterson goes on to call for a 'family strengths approach' to discover assets and resources which will enhance family members' capabilities and ensure that they are not overwhelmed. Stephanie had managed to overcome difficult teenage years and had formed a stable relationship with Liam. This was potentially a good foundation for family life. In addition, Liam's mother proved to be a supportive, well organised and a capable family resource to assist with Ami. This focus on strengths, resources and possible solutions rather than only on problems will be discussed again in Chapter 7.

As you can see and may have experienced, helping people like Stephanie and Liam with a very sick child or those who have to adapt to a changed lifestyle following illness or surgery can be very challenging. As well as changes in health behaviour and lifestyle, we may expect service users and carers to master physically complex tasks such as looking after a colostomy, Hickman catheter, caring for a tracheotomy or learning to live with a urinary catheter. Other families might have to find ways of coping with challenging behaviour, confusion or apathy. Whilst some may be able to adapt or even relish the challenge, for others it might take a great deal of patience on the part of professionals and all our skills in negotiation, teaching, motivation and support to help them succeed. We have to find the right time to introduce new skills and the receptivity of patient or carer will also influence the interactions we have with them (Euswas and Chick, 1999).

Caring and the challenges of compliance

One of the challenges that nurses may face is related to compliance with planned interventions or prescribed medication. Compliance implies that the person has agreed to follow and/ or act in accordance with expectations of what has been suggested, recommended or prescribed. However, if there is not agreement and clear understanding between professional and service users, compliance may not occur. Read the following observations of a visit by a student nurse and her mentor to Connie and consider the following:

+ What do you think the nurses would find when they repeated their visit to Connie?

+ What changes in approach might you have tried?

Case Study 5.6

'We were visiting Connie, a 65-year-old lady who is overweight and has a history of chronic venous leg ulcers and cardiovascular disease. She lives with her husband Fred who is in his 70s who looks after her and does most of the cooking and other housework. Connie spends most of her time watching television and doesn't get out much. Her leg ulcers weren't healing so the community nurse asked for help from the tissue viability nurse who visited Connie and advised the community nurse to redress them twice a week and use compression bandaging. Connie was very suspicious about whether this approach would help but both nurses went through the whys and wherefores and eventually she agreed. Two days later when we went in, we found that she'd taken all the bandages off and said that they were 'hot and uncomfortable' and 'making her short of breath'. Fred agreed with her. The community nurse told them that the bandages couldn't be causing the breathlessness and told Connie to persevere. She said that if she kept her legs elevated when she was sitting and tried to walk about a bit more it would help her circulation in general. The bandages were reapplied and we left Connie to try again.'

We expect that, like us, you doubted whether Connie would still have the bandages on her legs when the nurse visited her again. Bland (1999) provides good insights with her investigation into how people experience living with leg ulcers which might help us understand Connie's situation and guide our practice for a more effective outcome. Bland wanted to understand more about the pain and discomfort experienced and how people coped with it. This, as we have seen, is an important aspect of a caring attitude and she needed to get people's stories in order to understand why so many didn't comply with the treatment. She found that some people experienced major problems with wound odour and wound oozing which sometimes led to lack of compliance with wound management. To cope with the oozing, for example, people padded the wounds even more. Like Connie, some people found that particularly in hot weather the bandaging brought discomfort and was perceived as unsightly which led to them being removed. The smell also led to feelings of shame and embarrassment and also sometimes affected marriages by leading to a change in sleeping arrangements. They felt ashamed if others had to do the washing, e.g. of bed linen, and were reluctant to stay away from home because of this. There were feelings of being trapped in an imperfect body. Bland (1999) found that pain was often not assessed by the nurse so they were not able to enter into a true partnership with the patient since much of the information they needed to give good and effective care was missing. A caring and holistic approach, considering the psychological and the social impact of the effect of living with a leg ulcer, might have had dramatic effects on the outcome of the care provided. Bland went on to note that 'when the focus of the health professional is on wound management and the focus of the patient is on minimising the impact of what appears to be a permanent condition so he or she can get on with life, compliance can become problematic for the patient' (Bland, 1999: 54). Bland stresses the importance of identifying what problems may be in the way of complying with treatments or health-related guidance and in Connie's case an acknowledgement and further exploration of the discomfort she was having might have led to a change in attitude on her part or an agreement about another course of action.

There were similar findings for Bollini et al. (2004) who investigated problems of adherence to treatments for people with mental illness and their families. They found some of the problems related to denial of illness, adverse reactions to treatment and lack of clarity about their condition and plans for the future. Forsyth (2007) found another problem concerning the emotional reactions of the nurses and their beliefs about people. He investigated the nature of the nurse–client relationship when an individual has complex problems such as those leading to a diagnosis of a borderline personality disorder (BPD). Engaging with these clients could bring feelings of anger and negativity in the nurse, who judged them as responsible for their own actions and dismissed their behaviour as attention-seeking.

There are parallels for this in other areas of nursing where individuals may be blamed or held responsible for their problems, e.g. those who are overweight, those with smoking- or alcohol-related diseases, or even those, like Connie, with non-healing leg ulcers. Forsyth (2007) stressed the need for reflection on practice so that we articulate and understand our emotions, indicating that this will help us to understand what might be standing in the way of our being able to identify the best ways to help clients. Learning from our emotions will be a theme in the next chapter.

Time to think back

The stories of Ami and Connie have illustrated the challenges of holistic care in practice and creating effective partnerships with carers and those receiving care. They have helped demonstrate that it requires a great deal of patient, skilled observation and ability to identify what problems may be in the way of complying with treatments or health-related guidance. Ami was at risk because she was vulnerable and her parents needed to develop not only the parenting skills necessary for any child but also those needed for the care of a child with disabilities. Her safety and protection were key areas of concern. This called for a multi-professional and multi-agency approach in order to focus not only on the multiple problems there were but also on the family strengths and resources available. Connie's story also demonstrated why equitable and effective partnerships with service users are essential.

Being out of step

People may feel themselves to be 'out of step' with health professionals and this may give rise to distressing ethical debates. Read Jasmine's story and consider what decision you think staff looking after her may have come to.

Case Study 5.7

Jasmine was 14 years old and had been discharged from hospital. She had been diagnosed at an early age with leukaemia and had been through a number of treatment regimes – the latest had been extensive and had left her and her family feeling negative and emotionally drained. It was apparent that the pressures of living with such an illness were having an increasing effect on Jasmine and her parents. Jasmine also had a 2-year-old brother, Thomas, whom she enjoyed looking after.

Jasmine made a decision that she no longer wanted to comply with medications and treatments but wanted to live the rest of her life at home with her family. Her parents believed that she had thought things through and made the decision and that there was nothing more they could do in persuading her to comply. Staff in the unit were unhappy and frustrated. They did not want to 'give up the fight' although it seemed that this is what Jasmine and her family wanted.

Although this is a difficult situation, it presents the kind of ethical dilemma you will come across throughout your career, and your academic work related to legal requirements, human rights and ethical theories and frameworks will help you consider these complex practice situations from different standpoints and see how they may be applied to everyday decision-making. These also underpin professional standards and the NMC Code of Conduct (2008) which, as a nurse, you are required to follow. To caring professionals, 'letting go' of Jasmine and letting her do as she wishes may seem uncaring, but you may also have thought that not doing so could be considered to be paternalistic in that staff may be at risk of trying to make decisions on behalf of Jasmine and her family.

In Jasmine's case, although there were some misgivings initially, medical and nursing staff did not try to challenge the family's decision but shared all the information available to them about the likely consequences of their action so that Jasmine and her family were able to make a well considered and informed choice. Jasmine was able to return home, supported by community staff, and live with her family in the last few months of her life. Jasmine did not want to endure any further treatments, she knew she would die, but made a clear decision that she wanted to do this peacefully at home with her loved ones. Maude and Hawley (2007) remind us that children (as long as they fully understand and are able to make an informed decision) have the same rights as adults. Staff were able to draw on a good relationship, built up over a number of years with both Jasmine and her family, to ensure any decision was well considered. By doing so they may have been guided by the four main principles used to guide ethical practice: autonomy, beneficence, justice and non-maleficence.

In health care, autonomy means that an individual has a right to make their own decisions, e.g. to consent to or refuse treatment. This requires open communication between staff and the patient/client so that they are able to 'deliberate rationally through various possible courses of actions without being impaired by lack of time, incomplete information, mental illness and/or impairment' (Newham and Hawley, 2007: 79). Jasmine had time, was informed of the consequences and was able, with her parents, to make a rational decision.

Beneficence means that action is in a patient's best interests – what is seen as beneficial, or good for the well-being of the individual. Providing information and continued support at home, helped staff to act in Jasmine's best interest in terms of what she and her family wanted.

Justice is acting in way which is fair and equal. Jasmine was given the opportunity to continue a pathway of treatment, as another person in her situation would be, but she chose to refuse it. She was not penalised or discriminated against because of this action but support and help continued.

Non-maleficence refers to 'doing no harm'. It covers not only a duty of care but also the need to avoid both actual harm and the risk of harm (Newham and Hawley, 2007). This could suggest that this principle was not met as without further treatment, her death could be hastened. However, another application of this principle would be to consider that more treatments would cause her suffering, pain and separation from her family.

We hope that this will help you to see that theories and frameworks can be very helpful. Caring does require critical analysis of difficult situations, particularly those that involve an ethical dilemma and for which we need to reflect on ethical and legal considerations if we are going to be better able to help patients and their families and safeguard ourselves. We need all the resources available to help us to do that and acquiring knowledge of principles such as those acquired from ethics will help us a great deal. To be caring means that we should ensure that we are open to new knowledge throughout our professional life. This is what we mean by life-long learning.

Some people may also feel isolated or out of step with professionals because of their condition. O'Loughlin (1999) found that people with chronic pain often felt lonely, isolated and fearful and might find themselves labelled as 'the chronic pain patient' with the covert assumption that the pain was 'in the head' and therefore not valid. She described the experience of a patient who had a psychiatric history and felt negative stereotyping occurred because of this. Some health care professionals she thought had the belief that her chronic pain originated from the mind and was therefore illegitimate. As a result she felt dismissed and not valued as a person. She also found there were difficulties for the family. One sufferer told her, 'My husband tells me that when you've got chronic pain, you are a chronic pain. He's not trying to be nasty. It's just that that's what it's like to live with someone who has pain all the time', (O'Loughlin, 1999: 134).

O'Loughlin found health care professionals generally had inadequate knowledge of the complexities and effects of living with chronic pain. Pharmacological interventions may be prescribed but she claimed that these might not be the answer if there are side effects which may lead to feelings of frustration and anger, and highlighted the need for a range of measures to assess and treat pain such as the more holistic approach taken within pain clinics. Caring for someone in pain means trying to understand it. According to Madjar (1999), pain relief depends on the experience being shared and so requires visibility – we need language to describe pain. People may try to keep it private and therefore invisible – they may try to protect others and to keep their composure. The nurse needs to help the patient to describe pain and to share with them in the control of that pain. Madjar (1999) related this to caring which she defined as paying close attention to human experience but noted that it requires knowledge, skill and sensitivity.

To think about

+ Can you thinks of anyone you have cared for who may have thought they were 'out of step' with professionals?
+ What did you do, or might you have done, to help them?

Nurses aren't miracle workers

Sometimes we have to come to terms with the fact that people may have different preoccupations, drives and motives and we may find it very difficult to divert them from what we see as risky or harmful behaviour. Marcus, a community psychiatric nurse, told us of his work with Brett, a 30-year-old man, with a fourteen-year history of substance dependency including injecting heroin into his groin. He also had a complex history. He had been treated for deep vein thrombosis, bloodborne infections and was hepatitis C positive. He had little contact with his family and few friends, with his main form of 'support' coming from his drug dealers.

Read the following account of Marcus's intervention with Brett and consider what aspects he might have wanted to reflect upon, both during and after the event.

Case Study 5.8

'I saw my nursing role as one of persuading Brett into treatment to reduce risks mainly around unsafe injecting. This was to be done by substitute prescribing of methadone and key work sessions around harm reduction.

Brett was always difficult to engage. He did not always keep to agreed times of appointments and continued to groin inject. On one occasion, he informed me that he had started taking solvents. I asked him what this was and he said it was Butane gas directly from the can. I was very concerned and told him about the increased risk that he was putting himself in. I tried to explore 'triggers' that he felt led him to use the gas and strongly reinforced how dangerous it was. He told me not to worry, that he would be OK. I tried to be realistic in what behaviour he might be expected to change as I knew this was the only way I could get him to listen to me. I suggested that, if he continued to use Butane in spite of the risks to himself, it was safer to inhale from a bag rather than directly from the can. I really felt that he had taken this on board. However, this was not the case as he was found dead a week later through inhaling from a can. I felt sad, angry with myself for not being able to prevent it but also very angry with him.'

Compare your considerations with ours

It was obvious to us that Marcus cared greatly about Brett but he had mixed feelings of anger and frustration as well as feelings of sadness. Perhaps he asked himself if he had been caring enough and he would have needed support which may have come in the form of clinical supervision or debriefing.

Marcus would have considered whether he had used the 'right' approach – and why he was angry and upset. However, it was important for him to reflect that he had drawn on ethical principles to guide his practice, e.g. he tried his best to listen and negotiate with Brett, provided information and a plan of action which he thought might be less risky (even though it was far from an 'ideal' solution). In doing so he was trying to avoid harm coming to Brett as much as he possibly could, given the complex circumstances.

As he failed to influence Brett, Marcus was disappointed with himself (and also with Brett) but we have to come to terms with the fact that we may not always succeed. Reflection can help us with this and we can draw on assistance from literature. According to Narayanasamy (1999), we can facilitate change in others but we should not assume responsibility for that change. Health behaviour is complex. A number of methods can be used to try to help those at risk to change their behaviour, but motivation and the nature and magnitude of the problems the individual faces will play a significant part (Morrison and Bennett, 2006).

Nurses often have very high expectations of themselves although many factors may stand in the way of what they see as 'perfect' practice. Marcus may have what Glasberg et al. (2007) describe as the 'troubled conscience' all health care workers may have when they feel they cannot provide the 'good' care they wish to give.

It is this kind of complex situation that is a problem for nurses as, as we have seen, professional achievement influences our evaluation of ourselves as caring nurses. Clouder (2005) argues that when student health professionals undergo practice placements, they meet challenges to themselves as caring people and undergo a transformation in their sense of identity. She suggests that 'caring is a 'threshold concept' because of the 'troublesome knowledge' with which students are confronted. For her, this means that when faced with the reality of practice students have to revise their thoughts about what they mean to be caring since not everyone can be cured or treated, some interventions may fail, some people may not respond to care or may refuse it. From our experience and as expressed in Marcus's story, it would seem that nurses have to do this in a thoughtful and reflective manner throughout their career, particularly given the number of ethical dilemmas which occur.

Sometimes, a situation we encounter helps to keep our feet on the ground. What do you think we can learn from the following?

Case Study 5.9

Peter is a 12-year-old boy who has to have a supra-pubic catheterisation every three to four hours. He has required this since he was a baby because without the catheter he cannot empty his bladder properly and there is a leakage of urine. The nurses in the community have worked with Peter and his family since he was very young. Their input has been varied and very substantial, ranging from catheterising Peter when he was too young to do it himself, to teaching his parents, and then Peter, how to catheterise, liaising with the school to assist with inclusion and confidentiality issues. The school were great and even had a school shower installed for him to discreetly use. None of his school peers knew of this catheterisation issue, so that was never a problem. The school, nursing staff, parents were all so supportive towards Peter and worked very well together to get everything sorted for him. When he was about 10 or 11 years old, Peter declared he was not bothered whether he was wet or dry. He would not catheterise himself and chose to wear an incontinence pad. Everyone tried to get Peter to change his mind. For example, at school he was reminded about the catheterisation when due, and of course the staff members were very discreet so that his peers did not know. The nurses did body image and self-esteem work and so on. This was to no avail and went on for well over a year. The multi-disciplinary team's anxiety was very high and the staff and Peter's parents were in despair, saying they just did not know what to do next. Eventually, Peter's psychologist told them that it was their problem and not Peter's and that until Peter wanted to conform there was little left to do. This did not seem to help anyone's anxiety or frustration!

Earlier this week Peter's mother phoned the nursing team both laughing and crying. She said, 'You will never believe this and I feel awful about what I said to Peter but it seems to have worked. Peter is now suddenly self-catheterising and is very proud of being clean and dry. I was so desperate and angry so I said to him, "Girls don't like dirty little boys like you".' That stopped him in his tracks and he has certainly changed his behaviour now. All of your hard work and that is what did the trick!

This story reiterates the points made earlier about the importance of timing and receptivity of the patient. Peter had reached a stage in his life where his appearance and the way he was perceived by others (especially girls) mattered to him. His mother, exasperated and frustrated, inadvertently pressed the right button!

The importance of continuity of care for carers

Sometimes thoughtless care can undo what has been achieved over a long period of time. Read Luke's account of his father's stay in hospital and consider what problems there were and the benefits which might have been gained from ensuring a better relationship with the relatives.

Case Study 5.10

'Following his severe stroke we worked really hard for three months to help Dad regain continence, he then went into a respite centre to allow my wife and I a long weekend. Just before we left we had a telephone call informing us that Dad had fallen and hurt his back. He was admitted to the local hospital and the consultant told him that he would remain there till we returned home. Dad told her he hadn't passed urine since his admission. Because the consultant knew our concerns about the length of time it had taken to get him continent, she asked the junior doctor to pass a catheter, drain the bladder and remove it.

On return from our weekend, Dad had been moved to another ward. We noticed a very, and I mean very, full catheter drainage bag alongside the bed. I was furious and went to see the nurse in charge. She informed me that the use of a catheter was standard practice and couldn't be taken out until the doctors did their rounds the next day.

The following morning, the registrar agreed to speak to us. In response to my protests that it had taken three months for Dad to regain continence, he said the catheter would be removed. On visiting in the evening Dad was sitting out in a chair. Although the catheter had been removed, he didn't know where the toilets were and was sitting in his sodden trousers. Nothing was recorded in the fluid balance sheets. A care assistant came to help clean and change Dad. When we visited the next day it was apparent that he was regressing. He was sodden again, so I took him to the bathroom to wash and change him. Dad then decided that he wanted to go for a walk and proceeded to walk to the ward exit. "I want to come home," he said. We saw the nurse in charge and explained our concerns. The next morning he was discharged. It took two months for him to regain continence to the level experienced before the re-catheterisation.'

Problems

+ Lack of co-ordination and continuity in care meant that decisions were not communicated and acted upon which made Luke feel as if all the care and continence promotion that the family had provided was disregarded.

+ In the second ward, catheterisation appeared to be 'routine' rather than a considered decision based on individual circumstances. Luke felt that hospital staff had taken the easy route. He told us, 'Catheters are easy to pass and do control incontinence, but at what price to the patient and carer?'

Reasons for a better relationship

+ Care did not begin and end with the professional input but was a continuum of care, with the major amount undertaken by Luke and his wife. Their views, and those of their father, should have been taken into account.

+ Luke's father did not feel cared for. He suffered loss of dignity, self-esteem and feelings of powerlessness. It is no wonder he wanted to go home. Once more he had to go through an intensive relearning process. His experience might also affect the way in which he viewed any professional help or hospitalisation in the future. Neither he nor his relatives had trust in the professional care they were receiving.

+ The fact that Luke and his wife needed respite care indicates that they may have found caring for their Dad tiring and at times demanding. If more attempts had been made in promoting continence, the impact of the hospitalisation might have been less stressful.

+ The lack of co-ordination with, and respect for, relatives may have resulted in long-reaching consequences if they then felt no longer able to cope – having an impact both economically and in terms of a greater need for resources in general.

Summary

In this chapter we have seen the importance and necessity of creating effective partnerships with carers and those receiving care. Holistic care is not easy within changing political, economic and social contexts but can be helped if we work closely with relatives and their families in identifying not only problems but also family strengths and resources. Recognition that, as professionals, we are often only one small part of a continuum of care will make us more alert to the importance of ensuring that we work with informal carers. Patient and carer participation in care evaluations, forums and services such as PALS all help to do this, but in everyday practice we must make sure we enter into effective dialogue with service users and their carers. Paying attention to what people say about their lived experiences of illness or disability, of providing care and being cared for, will help us to bring into effect the most important aspect, that of truly caring partnerships.

Looking forward

To develop our capacity to be caring in our care, we need to learn more about others and also about ourselves. In the next chapter we will focus on how we might use our emotions and learn from them.

Activity

One of the care indicators you will see at the end of this chapter refers to looking for and knowing about resources.

+ How do you keep up to date with all the changing government policies?
+ Do you help service users and carers to do this?
+ How can the evidence be used to help you attain some of the outcomes and proficiencies set out in your nursing programme? There are various resources which can help. Please see further reading at the end of the chapter.

Caring indicators

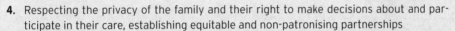

1. Helping someone to function at their optimum level
2. Helping to change a distressing situation into a manageable one
3. Helping someone to retain a sense of personal worth, acceptability and hope
4. Respecting the privacy of the family and their right to make decisions about and participate in their care, establishing equitable and non-patronising partnerships
5. Engage in effective multi-professional, multi-agency care, making patient and carers of central importance
6. Being alert to client 'readiness' by recognising the time to give supportive help and information
7. Not making assumptions but listening to what people, including children, say, paying attention to how they describe their situation and their lived experience
8. Understand and support carers in meeting competing demands
9. Give positive feedback to carers so they feel recognised and appreciated
10. Helping carers to look for and know about resources available
11. Recognising as professionals we are often part of a continuum of care
12. Caring is taking into account whole family needs and providing emotional support for them as required
13. Developing skills of negotiation, motivation, teaching and support to help informal carers succeed
14. Engaging in critical analysis of practice situations using resources, including academic, legal and ethical knowledge to help safeguard patients, families and ourselves
15. Willingness to engage in hard physical and emotional work
16. Being realistic - recognising you're not a miracle worker or angel - accepting that we may not always achieve what we want to achieve

Further reading

The Department of Health website on www.dh.gov.uk. In its publications section you will be able to keep up to date with government policies and guidelines and also information which will be useful for carers such as a booklet entitled *Information and Support for the Carers of People with Dementia*.

You can download a toolkit and supplementary resources which highlight good practice in involving people with dementia in service planning, delivery and evaluation. This has been developed with the help of patients and their carers and can be found at www.olderpeoplesmentalhealth.csip.org.uk (last accessed 27 January 2008). Click on the 'Visit the strengthening involvement pages'.

The Public Service website: www.direct.gov.uk
The Carers' website: www.carersuk.org
The Dementia Support Group website: www.dementialink.org
The Social Care Institute for Excllence website on www.scie.org.uk has quick and easy access to key research and policies and also ideas from practice.

References

Aggarwal, N, Vass, A, Minardi, H, Ward, R, Garfield, C and Cybyk, B (2003) People with dementia and their relatives: personal experiences of Alzheimer's and of the provision of care. *Journal of Psychiatric and Mental Health Nursing* **10**, 187-197.

Aldridge, J and Becker, S (2003) *Children Caring for Parents with Mental Illness: Perspectives of young carers, parents and professionals.* London: The Policy Press.

Bland, M (1999) *On living with leg ulcers*. In Madjar, I and Walton, J (eds) *Nursing and the Experience of Illness: Phenomenology in practice.* London and New York: Routledge.

Bollini, P, Tibaldi, G, Testa, C and Munizza, C (2004) Understanding treatment adherence in affective disorders: a qualitative study. *Journal of Psychiatric and Mental Health Nursing* **11**, 668-674.

Brouwer W, Van Excel, N A J, Van den Berg, B, Van den Bos, G A M and Koopmanschap, M A (2005) Process utility from providing informal care: the benefit of caring. *Health Policy* **74**, 85-99.

Clouder, L (2005) Caring as a 'threshold concept' transforming students in higher education into health (care) professionals. *Teaching in Higher Education* **10**, 505-517.

DoH (Department of Health) (2005) *Carers and Disabled Children Act 2000 and Carers (Equal Opportunities) Act 2004 Combined Policy.* London: The Stationery Office.

DoH (Department of Health) (2006) *Our Health, Our Care, Our Say.* London: The Stationery Office.

DoH (Department of Health) (2007) *New Deal for Carers*. London: The Stationery Office.

Euswas, P and Chick, N (1999) On caring and being cared for. In Madjar, I and Walton, J (eds) *Nursing and the Experience of Illness: Phenomenology in Practice.* London and New York: Routledge.

Forsyth, A (2007) The effects of diagnosis and non-compliance attributions on therapeutic alliance processes in adult acute psychiatric settings. *Journal of Psychiatric and Mental Health Nursing* **14**, 33–40.

Glasberg, A, Erikson, S and Norberg, A (2007) Burnout and 'stress of conscience' among health care personnel. *Journal of Advanced Nursing* **57**, 392–403.

Kitwood, T (1997) *Dementia Reconsidered – the Person comes First.* Buckingham: Open University Press.

Kitwood, T and Bredin, K (1992) *A* new approach to the evaluation of dementia care. *Journal of Advances in Health and Nursing and Nursing Care* **1**, 41–60.

Madjar, M (1999) *On inflicting and relieving pain.* In Madjar, I and Walton, J (eds) *Nursing and the Experience of Illness: Phenomenology in Practice.* London and New York: Routledge.

Maude, P and Hawley, G (2007) *Clients' and patients' rights and protecting the vulnerable.* In Hawley, G (ed) *Ethics in Clinical Practice.* Harlow: Pearson Education.

Morrison, V and Bennett, P (2006) *An Introduction to Health Psychology.* Harlow: Pearson Education.

Narayanasamy, A (1999) Learning spiritual dimensions of care from a historical perspective. *Nurse Education Today* **19**, 386–395.

Newham, N and Hawley, G (2007) The relationship of ethics to philosophy. In Hawley, G (ed) *Ethics in Clinical Practice.* Harlow: Pearson Education.

NMC (Nursing and Midwifery Council) (2008) *The Code: Standards of conduct, performance and ethics for nurses and midwives.* London: Nursing and Midwifery Council.

O'Loughlin, A (1999) On living with chronic pain. In Madjar, I and Walton, J (eds) *Nursing and the Experience of Illness: Phenomenology in practice.* London and New York: Routledge.

Patterson, J (2002) Understanding family resilience. *Journal of Clincial Psychology* **58**, 233–246.

Phillips, J, Bernard, M and Chittenden, M (2002) *Juggling Work and Care: The experiences of working carers of older adults.* London: The Policy Press.

Witton, M (2003) Support act. *Nursing Standard* **18**, 14–15.

Witucki-Brown, J, Chen, S, Mitchell, C and Province, A (2007) Help-seeking by older husbands caring for wives with dementia. *Journal of Advanced Nursing* **59**, 352–360.

Chapter 6
Learning from our emotions

LEARNING OBJECTIVES

By the end of this chapter you should have an understanding of how:

1. Accessing and analysing our emotions can help us to learn more about ourselves
2. Self-awareness and self-regard can influence our interactions with others and our potential to learn
3. Reflective strategies including the use of metaphors can increase our understanding of self and others
4. Developing our emotional intelligence can enhance our caring skills and influence our personal and professional development

Introduction

In this chapter we shall consider how we can learn more about ourselves by understanding our emotions and how we might use them to develop our capacity to be caring in our care. We will use examples from practice to discuss how reflection can increase our self-awareness and consider the ways in which we might be analytical about ourselves using metaphors and images to help us understand ourselves more. We will also explore the notion of emotional intelligence and its place in our professional development. We will discuss how all these aspects might help us to maintain and enhance caring approaches.

What our emotions do for us

It may sometimes seem as if our emotions are more of a hindrance than a help. They can cloud our judgement and our performance. We can be accused of being too emotional at times, in our everyday relationships as well as at work. It may mean we become too attached and upset by situations, react unthinkingly to what people say or do, or forget what we are supposed to be doing as we are so preoccupied with our own feelings. If we are to be caring, it is important to consider what our emotions tell us about ourselves and how we can best access them and learn from them.

In nursing, increasing our self-awareness is seen as an important requisite for effective interactions and critical reflection, but first of all it seems appropriate to think about what we mean by the self. Understanding ourselves is not an easy task as we are all complex individuals.

Stevens (1996) suggests that there are five aspects which help us understand what it means to be a person. It involves physical embodiment – we have a body with physiolgical sensations and responses which, as we know, may be prone to disease, stress and pain and which affect the way we perceive ourselves and are perceived by others. It also involves sub-jective experience as we use our ability to initiate thoughts and actions and make sense of our experience through our cognitive or thought processes. However, a third aspect is that we live in a social world so we are 'linked to others and exist in a social medium of meanings and customs' (Stevens, 1996: 16). This is a strong influence on our values, beliefs and preju-dices, as we are influenced by what we think is expected in our behaviour and attitudes (social norms). We know this is important in nursing, not only because of how we are socialised into it and perceive ourselves as nurses, but also because we are aware of the influence of cultural and religious beliefs on how patients feel about themselves and the ways in which they experience illness. Another set of influences on our self-perceptions is the likelihood of unconscious or hidden thoughts and feelings which may occur as a result of pre-vious experiences. Those adopting a psychodynamic approach, for example, emphasise the mechanisms we use to defend our ego (or sense of self) such as repression, denial and pro-jection, which we use in everyday life and may all act as barriers to self-knowledge. Lastly, Stevens highlights the important effect on us of the interrelationship of all of the above. In other words, he identifies the impact of a complex range of influencing factors on the way we perceive ourselves. This calls for a great deal of 'intelligence' so we are able to detect the influences of our own predispositions, characteristics, values and prejudices in our relation-ships with others if we are to be able to understand them and interact effectively with them. As you will see later in this chapter we will draw on an approach in which each individual is seen as an agent (in other words a manager) of their own social construction - this involves an active and changing process (Wetherall and Maybin, 1996).

A sense of personal identity, body image, role performance and self-esteem are all aspects of self-awareness (Kozier et al., 2008) and influence whether or not we have a positive view of our-selves. Our identity is a combination of physical and personality characteristics, values, beliefs and perceptions of our body image and our capabilities. These are all linked to how we regard our-selves in terms of self-esteem and role performance (e.g. as a mother, brother, friend, practitioner). Our self-concept changes as a result of development, our experiences, illness and stress. We have an image of ourselves as an 'ideal' person but all too often we fall short of this.

As students, you are going through a challenging period of learning and change. It is easy to focus on aspects you feel negative about but you also need to consider your strengths and how you can develop them further. This is because a positive self-concept is essential to our mental and physical health. It helps us to adapt and cope with change, in other words, to be more resilient. If we are positive about ourselves, we are also more likely to be able to help others (as long as we are honest and do not go to the other extreme of always excusing ourselves and only seeing ourselves in a favourable light). However, being self-aware and honest with ourselves is not easy. It requires courage, confidence, a certain degree of maturity and the support of others (Atkins, 2004). If we develop skills in self-analysis however, we will be able to evaluate our interactions, responses, behaviours and skills without feeling hopeless or worthless. This means applying the skills of critical analysis to ourselves – looking for a balanced judgement – highlighting the good points as well as the aspects we might need to develop or change. Thompson (2003: 133) emphasises that this process 'is not about self-indulgence or the emotional equivalent to navel-gazing but rather a more positive and constructive emphasis on self-awareness'.

We can develop self-awareness in a variety of ways but doing so takes time and energy. According to Thompson (2003) we can do this by adopting a more conscious and reflective approach as we go about our interactions with others and also by observing interactions between others. He suggests that the more we observe, concentrate and listen attentively, the more aware we can become and the more we can learn. We know that people with sensory deficits, hearing or visual difficulties, can develop extraordinary perceptual abilities in their other senses. There is therefore potential in all of us to develop our sensory capabilities. This will increase our ability to pick up cues or grasp meaning in encounters with others which is 'based on a capacity that involves the external senses as well as imagination' – an essential component of the art of nursing (Johnson, 1996: 251).

There are exercises designed to help us develop both physical and emotional self-awareness which may be undertaken as an individual, with a partner or as a member of a group (e.g. Thompson, 2002; Atkins, 2004). However, our everyday thinking or introspection also plays a large part in the way in which our self-image and self-knowledge evolve. If we go through a particularly emotional experience in practice we may go over and over in our minds how we behaved or others behaved and relive the feelings involved. Memories such as these can last for a very long time. Reflecting on our experiences can help us to analyse and change our perceptions. Some people find that keeping a personal reflective journal or diary is useful for this as it helps to externalise, articulate and review these feelings. Reflection therefore becomes the challenging aspect of memory. It makes us look again at what we have experienced and think about how we reacted. It helps to consider whether our input to a situation was effective by congratulating ourselves on what we think we did well but also noticing what gaps there might be in our knowledge or skills. This can provide us with the incentive to take any appropriate action needed for improvement and to consider what resources we might use to do this. This is why reflection has become so important in nursing. Duke (2004) has provided clear evidence of how reflection can become a vital and integral part of our ongoing professional life, outlining how it helped her to establish and develop her new role as a nurse consultant.

As we have said, there is a tendency for us, particularly when in a new situation, to focus on our limitations. There is a continual dialogue going on within us as we talk to ourselves about what is going on, what we make of it and how we should respond. Sometimes there may be feelings of panic as we try to find the best thing to say or do. There is an indication of the complexity of this inner speech in the following story written by a student nurse undertaking her first practice placement (Smith, 2003). Read her story and think about:

+ What phrases in the story are significant to help us understand her feelings?
+ What did she learn about herself?

> ## Case Study 6.1
>
> 'We pulled up in her car outside a house close to the sea. The community nurse told me we were visiting a lady in her early thirties, married with young children. She had breast cancer, had had treatment but secondaries had occurred in several parts of her body. She was terminally ill and receiving palliative care from the community nurse. A Macmillan nurse was also in attendance. Upon knocking at the door, I wondered what I might expect her to look and act like. Her sister opened the door, greeted us and directed us to the bedroom. Entering the bedroom, I noticed that the patient looked very depressed but she gave us a quick smile. My mentor engaged her in conversation. She answered with brief "yes" or "no" answers.
>
> After ten minutes of myself casually smiling, occasionally, my mentor informed me she was going back to the car. She had forgotten an enema. A sudden dread came over me! I was going to be left alone with this lady who I didn't know at all. What was I going to say? I quickly tried to think of something to say. The silence seemed awful. Maybe I should mention the weather. Oh no! That's silly - everyone talks about the weather. How boring! What did the weather matter to her, she wasn't going out anywhere she was so ill. Then I thought about asking her about Christmas, perhaps asking if her family were all prepared. Oh no, I thought - that's worse - she won't be expected to live that long. That might depress her even more.
>
> My mind went blank. I felt awful panicking inside. I quickly gazed round the room, then out of the window, groping for some inspiration. Then I finally saw it - the beautiful sea from her window. That seemed a safe thing to say I thought. I commented on the lovely view and how it reminded me of a house I used to live in, in Berwick upon Tweed, facing the sea. She smiled and said it was lovely. At that moment my mentor came back into the room and I sighed with relief. The nurse resumed her conversation and I never spoke again until it was time to say goodbye.

Compare your considerations with ours

We can learn a great deal by looking at her story closely and the language she used. She disclosed a great deal about herself - her thoughts and feelings. Her apprehension is reflected in her in the initial questioning about what a terminally ill patient might 'look and act like'. The story then goes on to provide a vivid insight into the way in which she searched for the 'right words' to say, and helps to understand the turmoil the student felt after being left on her own. You may have experienced this. Her use of phrases such as 'a sudden dread came over me', 'that would be silly' and the active 'groping for some inspiration', illustrate both her feelings of insecurity and the internal turmoil of her thoughts and feelings. She felt extremely vulnerable and she had to work hard to find the right words to say and yet appear calm. This is an example of emotional labour as described in previous chapters.

Initially, she was conscious of the need to feel part of the exchange between her mentor and the patient by 'casually smiling' but the responsibility shifted significantly when she was left alone. She is aware of the silence which she feels she must break and her consideration and consequent dismissal of what she saw as inappropriate topic areas add to her anxiety. She is also pleased that eventually she manages to find an answer and her relief is evident.

You may have found that, like us, you think that she told the story to demonstrate the difficulties associated with being left alone, and therefore responsible for communicating effectively with a terminally ill patient, an area of experience new to her. We followed her pathway of thinking and feelings as she told us details of her attempts to be caring and how she tried to avoid causing distress. She also indicated her relief when she found a solution to her problem. Overall, in spite of her misgivings, she seems pleased that she managed to find the 'right' words to say.

There are many ways in which her reflection on this experience would have helped increase her self-awareness and better understand what she could and did learn from it. Writing her story down, just as she recalled it, capturing her thoughts and feelings, provided a focus for further exploration. She could then have used a reflective model to guide her thoughts even further and analyse her behaviour. A variety of frameworks may be used to guide this, e.g. Gibbs's reflective cycle (Gibbs, 1988) or Johns's more structured approach (Johns, 2000).

In fact, the story was used as a focus for peer group discussion in which the student received positive support for the way in which she coped with the situation. It also provided an important opportunity for a group discussion about perceptions of what was 'appropriate' subject matter in conversing with dying patients, including the use of silence in communication. Further exploration of the literature about these areas helped all the students clarify and extend their learning by integrating practice and theory. The theory helped illuminate their practice.

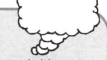

To think about

+ Write about a situation when you felt at a loss because you didn't know what to say or do (we all have them!). Write it as if you were writing a letter or an email to a close friend or an entry in your diary.
+ Look again at the language you use and underline phrases or words that show the emotions you felt. Then consider what you can learn from these about yourself and the way you respond in difficult situations.
+ You can deepen your analysis by linking issues which you discover with academic literature or theories, e.g. related to communication or the use of silence in interactions. This way you can see how what you have learned from your emotional responses has increased your understanding of issues arising in practice and has benefits for the way you manage your feelings and actions in the future.

We hope that the exercise helped you to describe, identify and analyse some of the thoughts and feelings which may occur as we undertake emotional work (or labour) within everyday practice. Becoming more self-aware has been described as the fundamental aspect of emotional intelligence (EI), which is the ability to recognise and use emotional information (Goleman, 1995; Orbach, 1999). McQueen (2004: 102) identifies the relevance of this to nursing, highlighting an important relationship between emotional intelligence and emotional labour, adding that 'the interpretation of emotional expression and intelligent response in the application of appropriate professional skills such as emotional work, empathy and counselling skills, can result in patients' emotional states being modified and anxiety ameliorated'. We have seen how this can occur in many of the case studies within this book (for example in the story of Harry and Rashida in Chapter 1).

The emotional part of learning

There is an emotional aspect to our learning which may not make sense immediately but some time after. In Chapter 4, we considered how our reactions to situations can be triggered by significant objects or events which make us think again about what we are seeing. The 'penny drops' and what we have experienced makes more sense. Consider the story about a visit to Frank by a student and her mentor and think about what we can learn from it.

Case Study 6.2

'On this particular day, I was out with the community nurse and we were visiting Frank who had a long history of alcohol abuse and self-neglect. The nurse warned me to expect some bad language and poor living conditions before we got there. It wasn't as bad as I expected. When we arrived there we found Frank sitting in a hole-ridden settee with springs poking through, wearing either his only or favourite suit by the look of it. The floor was quite littered with empty bottles and scrunched up cans. Frank was suffering from some kind of skin condition (I cannot remember what) due to his appalling diet or should I say lack of it. We treated his legs and got up to go. As we were leaving, the nurse asked him if he would have a shave before her next visit. I remember wondering why she had done this as I know there was no way he could actually get around to doing it. I didn't ask because I thought it would probably seem trivial to the nurse, but I always wanted to ask her if he did have that shave.

It wasn't until some months later that I thought about this again. I was doing some directed reading for once, on self-care. There was a question in the chapter asking you to think of an incident where there was a client with a lifestyle that was concerning and what the philosophy of care was when approaching this subject. Suddenly this memory sprung to mind and I realised what my mentor had been trying to achieve and how it related to what I had been reading. By *asking* this man to have a shave, not only was she encouraging him to take an interest in his lifestyle, she was giving him an option. This was much more ethical than just hanging in there and making him shave, either himself or doing it for him. No matter how good your intentions are for someone, this would surely undermine them and make them feel powerless and useless like a child. By giving this man an option, not only would he feel better himself for taking an interest in his hygiene, he would feel empowered as he was in control of how much care he received and who administered it. OK, this short-term boost probably wouldn't put him on the road back to recovery and make his life worth living again but it would show him that he is always capable of making things a little bit better ... step by step ... if only he chose to do so. ...'

Compare your considerations with ours

The story reminds us of the importance of the detail of description because it helps to begin the process of critical reflection. It can help if we look again at the student's story and try to précis it. She describes how a learning situation begins when she is reminded how a patient's condition and appearance are related to his lifestyle, although the situation does not seem as bad as she might have imagined. She questions why her mentor requested something that she thought was unlikely to happen (the shave), but does not ask for an explanation at the time since she thinks the nurse would probably think it was trivial. She recalls her question some time after by reading about self-care and realises what the nurse was trying to achieve by seeing a relationship between her experience and the literature. She is then able to attach value to the approach used by her mentor.

We can again look at the language she was using to get clues about what she was feeling. 'It wasn't until some months later' conveys the importance to her of the time gap between the incident and the reflection. The words 'suddenly this memory sprung to mind' provide an indication of the abrupt clarity with which she is then able to see the situation – the penny dropped. She emphasises the word 'asking' to underline her understanding of why the nurse gave Frank a choice. She seems pleased at being able to make the connection with theory and therefore able to explain to herself what happened, but the ending suggests her fear that effecting any change in the patient's lifestyle is likely to be a hard struggle.

Once more, this story provides an important message about how we learn about ourselves and the part reflection might play in that. It is an ongoing process as we try to learn from our experiences and link practice and theory. In this case the theory helped the student to understand an experience. Learning can be described as fitting the pieces of the jigsaw together. Sometimes it isn't until certain pieces are fitted together that we understand what the whole picture is about.

Learning from the language of metaphors

We used the metaphor of the jigsaw to help convey what we thought learning was all about. By encapsulating an image of feelings about an event, that image helps us to see things in a new light, in other words it helps to uncover hidden aspects. Like similes and images, metaphors are perhaps often thought of as a feature of literature, but are in reality very much part of our everyday life. The student, for example, in the story of Frank, talks about 'the penny dropping' and words 'springing to mind'. You may remember from your English lessons at school that a simile occurs when we use the word 'like' or 'as', such as when we ask, 'Does my skin look like a dried up prune from too much sun?' (we hope not!). We use metaphors as a figure of speech when we compare things, highlighting similarities, usually by saying one thing is another, e.g. 'She is a tower of strength'.

Throughout the ages and across civilisations, symbols, images and metaphors have been used in many ways as a form of communication about everyday life, as well as employed in a variety of spiritual, healing and religious practices. They are often a short-hand way of saying something and can help us make sense of our world by projecting rich and complex information that can appeal to a number of our senses – sight, hearing, smell and so on. Education, health care and social work, business and organisational management, are some of the communities that, in many different ways, recognise the power of similes, images and metaphors (Graham, 1995). They speak directly to our 'emotional mind'. For example, an advertiser may use a particular image as a way of engaging our unconscious associations, for example the picture of a person in a white coat holding a specific product might suggest, albeit at a subconscious level, that the product has scientific value and associations.

Sontag (1991) illustrates how military metaphors have, for a long time, been used in medicine as ways of expressing the processes and outcomes of disease, terms such as 'invasion of the body', 'war against disease' and 'victory over cancer' are some such metaphors. It is interesting, however, that Sontag (1991: 180) also warns about the use of metaphor in that it can 'powerfully contribute to the excommunicating and stigmatising of the ill'. She illustrates this by referring to a time when the AIDS virus was called the 'gay plague' and it was evident that the metaphor took on moralistic overtones. Patients use metaphors too. You may have heard some of them describing the phlebotomist as 'Dracula'. Madjar and Walton (1999: 9) highlight a vivid description from patients of staff 'harpooning' for blood when taking arterial gases and link this to a deeply felt experience which pictures both the weapon used and the action taken.

According to Watson (1999: 12), discussing their use within the context of nursing, 'It is important that the metaphors we employ or accept are made explicit so that we may better understand how they affect our seeing and being. They can be helpful or destructive. They can be unexpected or subtle parallels or analogies. They can encapsulate and put forward proposals or another way of looking at our reality or a given phenomenon.' Therefore by noticing the metaphors we use and which patients use, we can increase our understanding. Many people who have suffered from mental illness have tried to describe their experiences to others in terms of what others might find familiar. Roger who suffered from periods of depression was trying to tell his son what depression was like to help him understand. He said he felt like 'a deflated football – all the bounce has gone'. These images are very power-ful and help our understanding and therefore increase our empathy. They can also give an insight into our own perceptions, e.g. of growing older. In a collection of poems and writing, written at a creative writing session by older people and staff from a variety of services, get-ting older in our society was described as being separated from the rest of the community. Older people are like house plants that are only cared about when they need watering and then instead of being given a good long drink out comes the plant spray and all they get is the first watering of consideration.

As well as helping ourselves to gain more understanding, metaphors can also be a useful way of helping others, for example someone who is struggling to cope with extreme grief. Talking on a radio programme, a father described how, after the suicide of his son, he was helped by a priest who told him that it would seem as if he was always carrying a burden on his back but that, with experience, he would find different ways of carrying that burden. The use of the metaphor helped him see that the priest understood that he would never 'get over' his grief but gave him hope in being able to cope with it in the future.

The following story drawn from our own experience will, we hope, help you understand a little more about the potential for the use of metaphors in understanding, influencing and transforming practice. The case that follows was taken from a clinical supervision session which was used as a support strategy based on the premise that, in order to care for patients, nurses need to feel cared for themselves.

Case Study 6.3

'Our role was to help support the nurses on the nursing development unit (NDU) and the staff who wished to review their work to date and their professional role to determine what they thought was working well and where they wanted to 'go next' in their developmental process. We were acting as facilitators and knew that a number of authors suggest that the use of metaphors can help us think imaginatively about people and organisations, so we asked the staff if they would consider this. Although they thought this 'a bit academic' they agreed to try it out.

It was interesting, because metaphors (you have to listen for them) were used a great deal during our meetings. Some of the staff said that working in the nursing development unit was stressful because everyone seemed to be watching them; it was like 'working in a goldfish bowl' – because of the research funding the unit was receiving. The nurses were very conscious that "the paperwork was very demanding". They said they found it stressful because they believed totally in patient-centred, holistic care and a major theme of their discussions was that they really wanted to focus completely on "hands-on care to do their very best for each patient". It was difficult to get all of the paperwork done as this detracted from their caring role. "Paperwork is important: we need to protect ourselves and cover our backs."

The issue that came up time and time again was about the 'nursing boundaries', or rather lack of them. To give an example, at one of the meetings the discussion was led by a nurse who introduced the notion of 'difficult' patients and relatives. This nurse used the words: "They are difficult, you know those people who want you to dance to their tune". For example, one patient "refused to sleep at night, preferring to position themselves at the nursing desk and talk non-stop for ten hours to the night staff and then sleep during the day". Another nurse told of how a relative of an ill patient had continuously followed her to the canteen and talked to her about the patient all through her lunch and tea breaks. Staff said that they thought the hospital trust had not realised that nurses needed to get away from relatives when it allowed members of the public access to the canteen as a means of income generation. Someone noted that there are ways of avoiding these 'difficult' patients and relatives in the canteen and pointed to one of the group members saying, "You do it by walking fast and looking at the floor". This caused considerable amusement!

As facilitators of the session, we highlighted the keywords they were using – the metaphor "... those people who want you to dance to their tune". We then used extended metaphors as a way of helping the group examine various alternative scenarios.

"What would it be like if patients/relatives were to dance to your tune?"

"What would it be like for the patient/relatives to dance to their own tune and you ignored them?"

"What would it be like for nurses and patients/relatives to dance to their own tunes at the same time?"

"And if the tunes were totally different for nurse/patient/relative?"

This was followed by the question:

"Would it be possible to agree to a tune to which both nurse and patient/relative could dance: to make a joint melody?"'

It was by using these extended metaphors that these nurses came to acknowledge that they needed to learn how to cope with boundaries. There was recognition that all nurses sometimes have a misunderstanding that one's own self-needs must always be subordinated to the needs of others. Emotional and physical labour and issues related with 'burnout' (feeling physically and emotionally exhausted) were noted.

From this perspective they went on to explore ways of negotiating 'boundaries and limitations' that enabled a trusting, caring relationship characterised by power-sharing, empathy and mutuality in the contracting of boundaries. A variety of theoretical perspectives were introduced to the practitioners for them to further consider potential new ways of working. These included Berne's work on transaction analysis (Berne, 1968), which is about analysing and working with various communication styles – such as the nurturing and critical parent, adult and child transactions. Assertion skills and adult-to-adult styles of communication were discussed. The metaphors also provided direction for their reflections and opened up different possibilities for practice. Engaging in this reflective process seemed to help the nurses on the NDU gain a better understanding of some of their options for different ways of working. In other words it had the potential to help them to be emancipated (more open and less constrained in their thinking) and was likely to transform their ways of thinking and behaving in the future.

To think about

+ Think of metaphors which might describe the nature of a particular aspect of nursing practice. Time is an important element. Try to think of metaphors you could use which might describe your experience of this within practice.
+ Think of the metaphors a patient or client might use about this.

Compare your responses with those found in a research study. Smith (2003) described the metaphors students used. The most common metaphors and vivid descriptions related to time including notions of time flying or time standing still. Time was seen by both students and qualified nurses in their first two years following graduation as a valuable resource but also as a hard taskmaster. There were problems if time was wasted, if they were not given enough time to perform a task or if they took too long over one (as experienced by the graduate who compared unfavourably the length of time she took to give out medicines with her colleagues). There were descriptions of altered experience of time with 'time standing still' or 'dragging' and a minute 'seeming like an eternity' as students tried to think what to say 'to fill the silence' or when a newly qualified nurse waited for a more senior colleague to relieve her from an onerous responsibility. Time was a commodity which had to be managed and could be given (to patients) or taken (as 'time out' or 'five minutes for yourself'), providing an important way of coping with the job. There were 'not enough hours in the day' to do all they wanted to do, so participants felt guilty as they wanted to 'spend time' with someone and there was 'no time' available. The references to time increased as the students became more senior and following graduation. There were notions of 'running behind' and struggles to 'keep up' with everything. If the pace increased, participants could be 'flying around', 'running around in circles' or 'chasing your tail all day.'

You may have considered that sometimes, cut off from the normal flow of everyday life, time could move slowly for patients. Students in Smith's study described how patients had 'time on their hands' to worry and often had to play 'the waiting game'. One patient who had to deal with an unpredictable and life-threatening condition was described as a 'walking time bomb'. By thinking about the experience of patients in this way, we are able to 'connect' with their experiences in an empathetic way. This will help us to be more caring in our approaches. It can also help us to be more empathetic with ourselves and our colleagues.

You may think for example that you are the only one to be experiencing certain negative feelings but you may find parallels in the metaphors students in Smith's study used about their experiences of nursing practice. They sometimes 'felt on the outside' or even a 'nobody', as 'spare parts' or 'intruders' or 'easy targets'. They were worried about being 'thrown in at the deep end' or being 'out of their depth'. As they went through the programme, there was a requirement to do 'a balancing act' to cope with the 'tension of being a professional and remaining a person'. In the early stages following registration, most felt the stress of 'trying to find one's feet', 'being on the ball', being 'first in the firing line' and 'fitting in', but when help came or responsibility was taken on by someone else it felt as if 'a ton was lifted'. When they became the 'blue dress' and the 'buck stopped' they felt they should be able to cope with 'anything thrown your way'. In spite of the undoubted stress and 'problems taken home' there were also positive images of 'enjoying the buzz' and 'thriving on the new-found accountability.'

Metaphors also helped identify other emotional experiences of nursing as participants encountered situations which made them 'fume' or where they felt 'emotionally drained'. They were worried about 'going over the top', 'flying off the handle' or suffering from 'burnout'. They needed to stand back from situations and 'switch off' or 'become detached'. They were liable to go into 'overdrive' with 'the adrenaline rushes', 'live on the adrenaline' or conversely go onto 'automatic pilot'. There were images relating to extreme emotions such as 'tearing your hair out' or having your 'worst nightmares come true', signifying that they had to find a way of 'letting off steam' or 'sounding off' or they might 'bottle things up'. Fear could 'freeze solid in you' or an incident experienced could 'plague you for weeks'. Communications with colleagues could mean they felt they were 'struggling against a brick wall' or were 'between a rock and a hard place.' In their first year following qualification, they learned the importance of 'putting the ball into play' to bring about changes; 'keeping your eye on things'; of making 'on the spot decisions' and 'floating ideas' so they could 'move things forward'. Sharing these emotions through using metaphors helped them to empathise with common experiences and benefit from peer support – a key learning resource.

Emotional intelligence

We have emphasised the learning and benefits to be gained from sharing our emotional experiences with others and engaging in reflective activities. Like Duke (2004: 160), you may have discovered the power of reflection: 'the excitement and compelling nature of understanding something new or afresh, the richness of coming to know yourself'. We know that reflection is so widely used in nurse education since, as well as technical expertise based on evidence and organisational and management skills, nurses require self-awareness, motivation, self-regulation, empathy and skilfulness in relationships in order to practise effectively. These are the competencies which lie at the heart of what is called emotional intelligence and are essential for any situation where the focus is on interaction with others (people skills).

Goleman (1998) suggests that all those with higher emotional intelligence will be more successful at work and in their personal lives because of their high degree of self-awareness and ability to use emotional experiences to manage relationships more effectively and guide their behaviour. This is particularly relevant for nurses as they need to pay special attention to emotional cues of others, listen well, and respond to the needs of a variety of other people – patients, relatives and colleagues.

Freshwater and Stickley (2004: 93) underline this, reminding us that whilst we need to think rationally when undertaking technical nursing skills we also need to 'intuitively sense the needs and emotions of the person at the receiving end'. Developing emotional intelligence is therefore important not only in terms of the individual but also for organisations as it will affect the potential for teamwork, empowerment, creativity, patterns of communication, flexibility and the acceptance of diversity. It will have an effect on the ways in which we work with individual patients and their families and also on ways we work with colleagues.

It is not surprising therefore that there has been a great deal of interest in the usefulness of emotional intelligence in nursing, although Freshwater and Stickley (2004: 91) question the uncritical and unthinking application of it within nursing curricula, without 'fully grasping the entirety of its meaning and application'. Although they note the importance of the inter-dependence of rational and emotional intelligence, they suggest that much more needs to be done to promote stronger links between the two domains. They suggest that students need help throughout the curriculum to engage in learning which transforms or changes practice (in other words 'transformatory learning'). They suggest a range of activities which they con-sider to be useful for this such as self-inquiry, reflective discussion and writing, supportive supervision and mentorship, service user involvement in the planning and delivery of the course, use of art, drama, music, film and poetry. It might be helpful for you to consider what resources you have available to you as a student, and assess what helps you most in your emotional development, the growth of personal strengths and effective ways of responding not only to patients but also to patients' relatives and colleagues.

It is said that emotional competencies can be cultivated with the right practice if there is readiness to learn, motivation, effective support, good role modelling and clear, honest feed-back and guidance. A trusting and supportive environment in necessary and will be important for you to consider when you take on a mentoring role in the future. As well as learning from dialogue with critical friends and clinical supervisors, Duke (2004: 147), an experienced practi-tioner, also found it helpful to look for other strategies which helped her explore the meaning of her practice experiences as she describes how at times she became 'stuck in the reflective cycle'. She used poetry, metaphor and concept mapping to broaden and develop her skills. As we have seen, looking more closely at the way you describe your practice experience, e.g. by looking at the meaning of the metaphors you are using, may help you to discover more about yourself and the way you respond emotionally to practice situations.

To think about

We have described the usefulness of metaphors in helping us both to understand ourselves and others and to increase our emotional intelligence. We hope that what you have read will act as an impetus for you to continue to find ways of increasing this and of recognising the impact it has on your ability to care both for yourself and for others. You will find that changes will occur in the ways you both think about caring and act in the future as a result of learning from your emotions. It might be useful to ask yourself the following questions:

+ Are you able to identify various forms of support and resources which help you most?
+ Have you considered a range of strategies, such as the use of analysis of metaphors or the use of the creative approaches such as poetry or drama, to expand your knowledge of self and others?
+ Can you think of ways in which you changed (perhaps in the way in which you make judgements of situations and people or act) as a result of any reflective activity you have engaged in?
+ Has your learning about yourself resulted in some form of emancipation and transforma-tion? In other words has it freed you from ways of thinking and behaving that were not useful and increased your ability to cope with new or challenging situations in practice?

Reflecting on our possible selves

Whilst we have indicated the importance of being self-aware and highlighted some of the ways we might achieve this, we need to take into account that this journey is not straightforward and never ends as we don't remain static but change from day to day. Sometimes we feel 'spot on' and any problems encountered seem easily solved. However, all of us sometimes feel 'in the pits' and everything seems a struggle. We have different perceptions of ourselves and our capabilities at those times. How we view ourselves at any one particular time depends on what has happened before and what we believe is likely to occur in the future.

Markus and Nurius (1986) described the influence of our 'possible selves', suggesting that when we look at ourselves we make judgements of our value and worth, by taking account of a range of possible selves – what I was like, what I am like and what I might be like in the future. The importance of this is that it emphasises the fact that past and future possible selves (both negative and positive) can exert an influence on our present behaviour and feelings. 'Possible selves' 'represent individuals' ideas of what they might become, what they would like to become and what they are afraid of becoming' (Markus and Nurius, 1986: 954). They are important because all of these 'possible selves' act as motivating factors for our behaviour (influencing approaches and avoidance strategies). For example, a student who finds calculations difficult and is frightened of looking foolish might avoid assisting with the administration of medications. Rationally, there is no need to feel foolish because we all find some aspects of our work easier than others and the fear that we might have of others discovering our 'deficiencies' might lead to us missing out on an opportunity to learn.

The mixture of perceptions of 'possible selves' would seem particularly relevant to you as a student as you are engaged at a time of immense learning and personal change. Reflection can help you in that any ambiguities, tensions and judgements, associated with changing self-image and therefore self-esteem, can be accessed and utilised to influence the way you think about yourself. We often fear the worst about ourselves, and recognising irrational fears and building up our self-confidence is important. You may find that if you keep a personal diary in which you reflect honestly on your experiences, you can uncover the range of images and irrational thoughts you have about yourself.

Katrina found her first job in a nursing home following registration quite challenging. Read her entry in a reflective journal and think about how the emotions related to her 'possible selves' influenced her self-concept and self-esteem.

Case Study 6.4

'It was only my third shift working at the nursing home. I was on early shift and I was still not used to the routine and the residents' names. Upon arriving at work, I was horrified to discover that the charge nurse (my preceptor) had just phoned in sick and I was to be the only qualified nurse on duty with three health care assistants. The night staff gave a quick handover to us all, most of the names meant nothing to me, I couldn't put a face to a name. Instead of listening at handover, I felt myself shift into thinking about doing the drugs myself. Then on to emergency situations, there was no resuscitation team here. Hospital seems to be very safe, there are always plenty of people to ask. Here I felt isolated. I questioned my first aid skills and wished that I had done a first aid course; perhaps I'd feel more confident now.

The night staff left and the keys were passed on to me. Those all-important keys. I had a strong feeling of nausea. I allocated the work and we started to get the residents up, working as quickly as we could. I was constantly thinking to myself, "Please don't let anything happen, I'm just not ready." I felt as though I needed more time. At break I just couldn't eat anything, I felt sick and on edge. The shift passed quickly without any incidents and when the late-duty staff nurse came on, I felt relieved and it was with great joy that I passed those 'keys' over to him. I felt as if a ton had been lifted off my back.

Later, I reflected on my day and I felt angry that I could be left without knowing the residents or the routine. But after all, the health care assistants knew them well. My charge nurse could not help being ill and should anything have occurred, I'm sure common sense would have taken over. I felt really isolated and have realised that nursing homes are now not the easy option that they are portrayed to be but I know I am capable of coping'.

Compare your considerations with ours

Katrina's story provides a powerful image of the impact of a trajectory (journey) of anxiety throughout a shift as she felt the need to prove herself capable and sensed her inadequacies. We can see that her anxiety mounts as the story unfolds until the keys are taken away and the weight of responsibility lifts. She then questions her response as to who was to blame for the circumstances and reassures herself with the knowledge that nothing did go wrong, and if it had, it would probably have been OK anyway.

The telling of the story led to a reassessment of what she perceived she was like. Retelling how she performed in an extremely stressful situation helped her to articulate how she managed to survive, in spite of an early negative view of her own ability which affected her badly. Telling the story had the potential of helping her to overcome her anxieties by making her more aware of her capabilities. It was a story about overcoming adversity and building up her confidence in her ability.

We can see how her exploration of her 'possible selves' influenced her. She redefined herself – by considering what she was like in the past when she had support within a hospital setting, what she was like now (her inexperience and lack of familiarity made her doubt her ability) and what she might be like in the future (during the experience she thought it might all go wrong but by the end she was able to be more confident about the way she had coped and what she was capable of in the future).

It is not known whether Katrina reflected on this situation with her preceptor but it is likely that this might have led on to a clear identification of her learning needs (e.g. concerning emergency situations, giving medications, safety aspects, line management responsibilities and referrals) and also for gaining more reassurance concerning the strengths of her performance. It can be seen, however, that simply by telling the story she had begun the process in which a negative self-image was transformed into one in which she was beginning to see herself in a more positive light. If you do keep a reflective diary you will be able to see changes in the way you perceive yourself.

We have seen other evidence of this recognition of the transformation to a 'capable self' through experience (enhanced by positive feedback). A student described how she coped with (i.e. responded to, initiated the procedure for and managed) an unexpected cardiac arrest. She compared this with her previous 'nervous' self, and was confident that she would continue to be more confident and capable in the future.

Time to think back

Caring for yourself means recognising feelings which may be detrimental to you so that you are then able to respond in a useful way. As we have said, if you are over-come with feelings of inadequacy you are likely to give much greater emphasis to deficiencies in your performance than if you have a positive self-image. However, if you articulate your feelings you will be better able to accept and learn from them. Can you can recognise the influence of possible selves? As we have seen, they may be accessed through paying attention to your internal conversations or by writing down how you feel about a given situation.

Articulating and accepting our feelings

Carrie, a newly qualified nurse, found writing her feelings down about a complex situation raised questions that she needed to answer. Read the following account and consider the questions that it might have raised for Carrie.

Case Study 6.5

'Being a qualified staff nurse, you automatically think that the role/title in itself allows you to be knowledgeable, responsible and able to cope with any situation put before you. Not so. Working in intensive care, there are many situations which you (staff nurse) are supposed to deal with effi-ciently and maturely without letting personal feelings becoming involved. One incident occurred when I was looking after a sick patient and basically the decision was made to turn off all the life support. Simple. No, I felt as if I couldn't, wouldn't, be able to. After all, I'm only me, young enough to be this patient's daughter. Yet I was advising his wife, comforting the other relatives and nursing this dying patient in a very mature, responsible, staff nurse way. All the time I simply wanted to say - stop! Try again with this patient - don't let him die, as I can't handle this! Yet as a staff nurse you have to, regardless of your feelings or the person you are. Anyway the shift ended, relatives comforted, paperwork sorted, patient continuously nursed until 'his final hour'.

I've been told that, in time, you learn to accept it, accept situations more effectively and eventu-ally go home thinking, I've done a good job today. But that comes with experience. I'll let you know'.

Compare your considerations with ours

+ Is it rational for Carrie to think that 'being a qualified staff nurse, you automatically think that the role/title in itself allows you to be knowledgeable, responsible and able to cope with any situation put before you'?

+ Is she right in thinking that as a staff nurse you should be able to cope with situations without letting personal feelings become involved?

Carrie seems to be questioning whether she is mature enough to cope with the situation. Carrie should ask herself whether she has learned to manage her feelings about death. She might also ask herself to think about what constitutes doing a good job. We think she has unrealistic expectations of what might be expected of her as a newly qualified staff nurse. This notion of a perfect 'possible self' may have begun as a student. She feels she is 'acting' a staff nurse role but her emotions have overtaken her.

The significance of Carrie's story appears to lie in her reaction to the decision to turn off a life support machine and the action of doing so. There is no debate, however, over whether this is right or wrong for the patient (this would have been a team and family decision) but she concentrates on how the action affects her. She appears to be concerned that she has felt ill-equipped to deal with the event because of her inexperience and also personal misgivings – she doesn't want the patient to die. However, she is reinforcing her view that she has overtly supported the decision, by letting the routine take over and acting in a 'staff nurse way' by 'comforting the relatives' and providing care 'until the final hour'.

Carrie is viewing the decision from a personal viewpoint. It appears that she is finding it difficult to deal with the finality associated with the decision. She is indicating that she is unable to be objective and detached in a situation like this (which to her would be a sign of having 'done a good job') and is presenting an image of herself as young, emotional and inexperienced. This is reinforced by making comparisons of the patient as parent and herself as a child. At the end, however, there is an element of doubt that these feelings will continue and the possibility that there will be changes with experience is raised. However, when she reviews the situation with help she might be able to look at the reasons for her fears, e.g. her own or feared losses or death.

Carrie has used the story as a means of expressing her emotional feelings yet to be resolved. Talking this situation over with somebody else, particularly if she had written it down in such detail, would help her think again about her strengths and areas for further development. She could also question whether a caring nurse can remain so whilst being part of 'calculated and detached' decisions. It would seem that in managing her emotions (emotional labour) and putting the needs of the patients and family first, she was fulfilling a caring role.

Accepting our shadow side

Like Carrie, we are all fearful and upset at times and may also experience other feelings such as anger, annoyance, envy, competition, indignation, antagonism and bitterness. We all have a tendency to display what the psychoanalyst Jung (1966) called our 'shadow side'. However, he believed that it was important to find out about, accept and learn from this because of all the potential it has for personal growth.

Consider the following incident written by Maylin, a second year student nurse, and think about whether you have experienced similar feelings.

Case Study 6.6

'We visited Dawn, suffering from terminal cancer, in her home. During the visit we were to help her out of bed and put on a TENS machine to relieve the pain. I started to help my mentor put the machine on. To Dawn everything we did was 'totally wrong and in the wrong bloody order'.

Afterwards we discussed the visit and my mentor said that Dawn had been visited by another community nurse for months and probably didn't like the change. At the time of the incident I felt quite annoyed and frustrated at Dawn's attitude. When I had time to think about it, I felt disgusted with myself since she was in a lot of pain and probably did not have long to live. The most demanding thing was to hide my anger and, although I did not say anything to her, I think that she might have realised that we were both annoyed at her.

I think that this is important to reflect on since it showed me that sometimes it can be very difficult to cover up your feelings and care for someone. I thought that Dawn had made me feel angry and frustrated as nothing we did seemed right. However, as my mentor pointed out, Dawn might have been using angry behaviour to cover up her fear and feelings of insecurity. This helped me to realise that if I get the 'wrong feelings' about a patient, a useful coping mechanism might be to accept that we don't really know what is going on in a patient's life.'

So-called negative emotions we feel are often not openly discussed and critically explored. Perhaps this is so especially in our place of work, but that does not mean they are not present. As we saw in Chapter 3, angry patients, those who are perceived as behaving badly and ungrateful and demanding, can be unpopular with nurses and this can affect the care they receive. It is relatively easy to feel compassionate when confronted directly with the others' suffering, but we can feel threatened and disillusioned when faced with an angry patient or relative, because when someone gets angry with us we might get angry in return. We need to acknowledge and manage this. Emotions become threatening the moment they threaten to disrupt our calm and our emotional balance.

We may learn a lot about ourselves by reflecting on aspects of patients' behaviour that we find most difficult. This calls for a sort of detective work. It requires self-awareness, such as finding out why, how and when we are at our most vulnerable since different experiences and people affect us all in different ways. Acknowledging what irritates, hurts or annoys us most about other people has the potential to help us to have a greater insight into our personal shadow side, which otherwise can remain hidden. This means that when the patient's behaviour is difficult for us to address we do not see ourselves as a victim, nor do we view ourselves as superior.

Summary

In this chapter we have focused on what it means to be self-aware. We used examples from practice to discuss how reflection can increase our self-awareness and considered the ways in which we might be analytical about ourselves by using metaphors and images to help us understand more about ourselves and others. We also explored the notion of emotional intelligence and its place in our professional development, including competencies such as self-awareness, motivation, self-regulation, empathy and skilfulness in relationships. We stressed the importance of finding ways of developing these aspects if we are to maintain and enhance caring approaches.

We emphasised the role of reflection in increasing our self-awareness. When a strong emotional reaction has occurred it is important to reflect on the situation after the event, away from what Eraut (1994) describes as the 'hot action' where responses and demands in practice can be quite problematic. Sometimes our reflections can be the result of a sudden 'penny dropping' when our understanding takes on a new meaning or we are able to synthesise or integrate our learning experiences. We have also learned that reflection helps us uncover other important influences on our self-image; the impact of our beliefs about how we were in the past or might be in the future and on what we are like now (the notion of our 'possible selves'). Recognising ourselves as changing and developing leads to our realising the importance of understanding our ontological knowledge (what we 'are' – our 'being') as well as our epistemological knowledge (what we 'know').

Looking forward

Caring for ourselves is important if we are to fulfil our potential and be caring towards others. A better understanding of what makes us stressed and how we might manage this will help us to learn how to take better care of ourselves and develop emotional resilience to overcome some of the challenges we face. In the next chapter we will consider this and also discuss how consideration of our strengths and resources can help us achieve our goals.

Activity

Consider your personal professional development. Next time you begin a practice, record or write down your feelings about yourself – how you felt at the end of the first week (no holds barred – it's for your eyes only). Do it again half way through, and at the very end of the placement review once more how you feel about yourself. Listen to or read your entries and see what you can learn about yourself in relation to past, present and your future possible nursing self.

Caring indicators

1. Recognising and using the emotional aspect of learning including discussion and explorations of our negative emotions
2. Paying attention to, accepting and responding to emotional cues in self and others
3. Recognising our irrational and our unrealistic thoughts
4. Recognising our 'shadow side'
5. Using various reflective techniques and strategies to increase awareness of self and others, e.g. by using journals, metaphors in order to describe or identify, analyse thoughts and feelings, and transform practice
6. Helping others to adapt and cope with change

7. Learning from our emotions and developing emotional intelligence and emotional competency (self-awareness, motivation, self-regulation, empathy and skilfulness in relationships)

8. Promoting and developing positive self-concept for emotional and physical health in self and others

9. Becoming increasingly aware of and acknowledging our capabilities and our areas for further development

10. Recognising that what we may think we might be like in the future (our 'possible selves') can be either motivational or based on hidden fears

References

Atkins, S (2004) Developing underlying skills in the move towards reflective practice. In Bulman, C and Schutz, S (eds) *Reflective Practice in Nursing.* Oxford: Blackwell.

Berne, E (1968) *Games People Play.* Harmondsworth: Penguin.

Duke, S (2004) When reflection becomes a cul-de-sac: strategies to find the focus and move on. In Bulman C and Schutz S (eds) *Reflective Practice in Nursing.* Oxford: Blackwell.

Eraut, M (1994) *Developing Professional Knowledge and Competence.* London: Falmer Press.

Freshwater, D and Stickley, T (2004) The heart of the art: emotional intelligence in nurse education. *Nursing Inquiry* **11**, 91–98.

Gibbs, G (1988) *Learning and Doing: A Guide to Teaching and Learning Methods.* Oxford: Oxford Polytechnic.

Goleman, D (1995) *Emotional Intelligence.* London: Bloomsbury Publishing.

Goleman, D (1998) *Working with Emotional Intelligence.* London: Bloomsbury Publishing.

Graham, H (1995) *Mental Imagery in Health Care: An introduction to therapeutic practice.* London: Chapman & Hall.

Johns, C (2000) *Becoming a Reflective Practitioner: A reflective and holistic approach to clinical nursing practice development and clinical supervision.* Oxford: Blackwell Science.

Johnson, J (1996) *A Dialectical Examination of Nursing Art.* In Kenney, J (ed) *Philosophical and Theoretical Perspectives for Advanced Nursing Practice.* London: Jones & Barlett Publishers.

Jung, C (1966) *Modern Man in Search of a Soul.* London: Routledge & Kegan Paul.

Kozier, B, Erb, G, Berman, A, Snyder, S, Lake, R and Harvey, S (2008) *Fundamentals of Nursing: Concepts, Process and Practice.* Harlow: Pearson Education.

Madjar, I and Walton, J (1999) *Nursing and the Experience of Illness: Phenomenology in practice.* London and New York: Routledge.

Markus, H and Nurius, P (1986) Possible selves. *American Psychologist* **41**, 954–969.

McQueen, A (2004) Emotional intelligence in nursing work. *Journal of Advanced Nursing* **47**, 101–108.

Orbach, S (1999) *Towards Emotional Literacy.* London: Virago.

Smith, A (2003) *Learning about Reflection.* PhD thesis, Northumbria University, Newcastle upon Tyne.

Sontag, S (1991) *Illness as Metaphor.* London: Penguin.

Stevens, R (1996) *Understanding the Self.* London: Sage.

Thompson, N (2002) *People Skills.* Basingstoke: Palgrave Macmillan.

Thompson, N (2003) *Communication and Language.* Basingstoke: Palgrave Macmillan.

Watson, J (1999) *Postmodern Nursing and Beyond.* London: Churchill Livingstone.

Wetherall, M and Maybin, J (1996) The distributed self: a social constructionist perspective. In Stevens, R (ed) *Understanding the Self.* London: Sage.

Chapter 7

Surviving and developing by caring for yourself in order to care for others

LEARNING OBJECTIVES

By the end of this chapter you should have an understanding of:

1. Ways of learning to care for ourselves so we are better able to care for others

2. Ways of recognising, avoiding and managing stress so we can increase our emotional resilience

3. The importance of building on strengths and resources using a solution-focused approach which could be useful for extending our own capacity and that of families and carers

4. The ways in which we can extend our ability to care for ourselves and others through utilising our creativity and 'spirituality'

Introduction

As we have found, although stress is a part of everyday practice, the ability of some students and qualified nurses to care is diminished if they become overwhelmed with personal and professional issues, including unrealistic expectations of themselves. Caring for ourselves is important if we are to fulfil our potential, including finding the most effective ways in which we can care for others. A better understanding of what makes us stressed and how we might manage this will help us to learn how to take better care of ourselves and develop emotional resilience to overcome some of the challenges we face. In this chapter we will consider these issues and also discuss how our strengths and resources can help us achieve our goals. We shall use an example of a solution-focused approach to see how this strategy might help us.

Looking after yourself

Do you ever go home from your work placement feeling absolutely exhausted emotionally as well as physically. Every student nurse experiences stress. This can be a great motivator (for example it may help you to get your assignments finished and ready to hand in on time!) but it can also have an adverse impact on your physical, psychological and social health as you will have discovered from your study of the effects of stress on patients. There are indicators of the beneficial aspects of stress (eustress), such as speedier reaction times and the ability to focus attention on the specific situation. If we are in distress, however, there are negative indicators such as lack of self-esteem, short temper, negative attitudes, and coping mechanisms which may cause us harm, for example smoking and drinking. Stress is a subjective experience arising from individual perceptions and there are many perceived sources of stress (Kozier et al., 2008).

A better understanding of what makes us stressed and how we develop our own particular positive coping mechanisms will help us to learn how to take better care of ourselves. If we do so, we will be more competent in caring for others and will have satisfaction in a job well done which in turn can increase our self-esteem. However, Goleman (1999) says that 'empathy distress' is common for those who are in the helping professions, as they continuously have to cope in extreme circumstances and may have to deal with people in unpleasant moods. We therefore have to learn to be emotionally competent and not only be aware of our feelings but also be capable of not becoming weighed down by resentment, disillusionment and antagonism.

Covey (1999: 287) highlighted the importance of giving ourselves time for renewal. He used the following story to illustrate this:

> 'Suppose you were to come across someone in a wood working feverishly to saw down a tree. "What are you doing?" you ask.
>
> "Can't you see?" comes the impatient reply. "I'm sawing down this tree."
>
> "You look exhausted!" you exclaim. "How long have you been at it?"
>
> "Over five hours." he returns, "and I'm beat! This is hard work."
>
> "Well, why don't you take a break for a few minutes and sharpen that saw?" you inquire. "I'm sure it would go a lot faster."
>
> "I don't have time to sharpen the saw," the man says emphatically, "I'm too busy sawing."'

We often feel too busy to stop but may realise that this is not an effective way of trying to cope with situations. We were reminded of this by a group of ward managers who were engaged in a series of group reflective sessions so that they could share experiences and learn from and support each other. During a winter bed crisis when they were extremely busy, we suggested that they might want to cancel the next session. Back came the reply, 'It's when we're so busy that we need it most.'

Work stress, and its effects, is a serious health issue. As you may have learned in your study of its effects on patients, stress can have severe physical, psychological, social and spiritual effects and many illnesses are either caused or aggravated by stress. In addition Wicks (2006: 4) suggests that 'the pressure that results from the reaching out to others in need, is a constant and continuous reality in medicine, nursing and allied health' and leads to what he describes as secondary stress. Other factors such as colleague relationships, limited resources, organisational change and pressures also play an important part (Edward and Hercelinskyj, 2007).

You may be aware that severe and cumulative stress brought about by emotional or physical exhaustion can lead to a complex syndrome known as 'burnout'. This is found in people who work in numerous public service occupations including nursing. Signs of burnout include chronic fatigue and exhaustion, anger, cynicism, negativity, depression, feelings of helplessness and hopelessness and physical effects such as insomnia, headaches, weight loss or gain. There are also reports of an increased likelihood of risk taking (Edward and Hercelinskyj, 2007).

Goleman (1999: 288) claims that only a few organisations address the degree to which they themselves create stress and more usually blame the victims of burnout as if it were entirely the individual's defect. He cites a study to make his point about the relationship between burnout amongst nurses and patient satisfaction. 'In a large medical centre, the extent to which nurses on inpatient units had classical burnout symptoms like cynicism, exhaustion and frustration with working conditions correlated with patients' reports of dissatisfaction with their hospital stay. The more content nurses were with their jobs, the better patients rated their medical care.'

We therefore need to look for ways in which we can prevent undue stress or burnout happening, not only for ourselves but also because of the effects it will have on the ways in which we are able to care for others and relate to our families, friends and colleagues. In addition, one person's stress seems to be 'catching' and may induce stress in others leading to what Wicks (2006) describes as 'burnout contagion' and can therefore have a negative impact on the effective functioning of teams or organisations. An important aspect of leadership is to recognise early indications of this, determine the causes and find ways in which to change the culture into one in which people feel valued and have a shared sense of purpose and which is therefore more conducive to working in harmony and efficiency.

The second year 'blues' and the final year panic

As nurse teachers we have found that there seem to be specific periods when student nurses experience particular despondency and distress. Once the initial 'honeymoon' period within the first year is over and the initial excitement about beginning a new career has waned, students are faced with having to cope with the reality of practice and try to balance work, life and intensive academic demands. This is the time when students sometimes wonder if nursing is the right profession for them and they undergo what is known colloquially as the second year blues. It is often their friends or a skilled mentor who helps them to get over their misgivings.

For example, consider the case study below (cited in Smith, 2003: 237) written by a student at the end of her first year.

Case Study 7.1

'A patient expressed his concerns and anxieties to me about not receiving any information at all about why he could not go home as he felt perfectly well. Several times I told qualified staff about how the patient was feeling and how he was worried about not knowing what was happening. All they could tell him was that they were waiting for the results of the X-rays. This left him very frustrated. Maybe I was wrong in doing so, but I told him he should perhaps ask the consultant next time he came onto the ward as to why he had not been told anything.

The next day the consultant came onto the ward to see another patient and once again the patient came to see me and voiced his frustration. I told him that he should tell the consultant about how he felt when he passed. He seemed very hesitant and anxious so I stood by him as the consultant came by. The patient stood up and began to explain how he had not been told anything. The consultant interrupted and told him he had only been on the ward for a couple of days and that he would get a junior doctor to see him and walked off. During this brief interaction the consultant only made eye contact with the patient twice, and the rest of the time kept his head down and spoke as if to the patient's slippers. The patient was left standing open-mouthed. I will never forget the look on his face. He walked back to his bed shaking his head. I felt guilty as I was the one who had encouraged him to ask.'

It would be easy to focus blame on the consultant for not communicating well with the patient and this may well have been a cause for concern and needing further exploration. However, for the patient the most important thing would be to consider how best to relieve his obvious anxiety. The student had a role in conveying again the patient's concerns to her mentor or ward manager so that he could be seen as soon as possible. This situation made the student think again about her role and she felt despondent because she thought she was doing what was right in helping the patient in self-advocacy. She even showed her solidarity by standing close by him thus offering him emotional support. When her strategy for helping failed, she felt responsible and doubted her value.

This kind of incident which causes irritation and frustration is important as it can contribute to the build-up of stress. However, there are less likely to be problems associated with stress, even in pressurised situations, if the value or importance of the work is recognised. Ongoing stress is related to how it is perceived by us and by others (Wilkes, 2002). Individuals who see the relevance and value of the work they are undertaking, have the ability to 'bounce back' when meeting challenges or adversity and are less likely to experience emotional exhaustion (Glasberg et al., 2007).

The reality of, and challenges of, practice may mean our having to come to terms with a working environment which can be both rewarding and exhilarating but at other times hostile and difficult. It is easy for our attention to focus on the negative particularly at the times when we feel physically and emotionally exhausted. This might account for the second year 'dip' and also for the panic just before registration when students are undertaking the final practice placement. This can be a particularly stressful time as students struggle to meet important academic requirements and as the realisation of what it might mean to be a qualified nurse dawns. Knowing that other students experience these 'dips' should help by making you feel that you are not alone. On the other hand, you may have experienced 'stress contagion' within your peer group when one person's fears and grievances are 'caught' and influence the ways in which all members of your group feel, think and act.

Some ways of thinking appear to block other more positive thoughts and make it difficult for us to move on and overcome negativity. We become overly pessimistic and there is a tendency to blame others for our feelings and situations. It is obvious that in life we may not always be treated fairly and that things can happen which are sad, frustrating, unfair and even disastrous. Whilst it is important to acknowledge the problem and analyse why we are upset, angry or disappointed about a workplace situation, it is not helpful to spend too much time on discussions about who or what was to blame. This can inflame our dissatisfaction so it is better to look for ways in which we can overcome our anxieties, cope with and handle difficult situations.

Abraham (2004) emphasises the value of developing emotional resilience which he describes as 'flexible optimism'. Instead of engaging in fault-finding, individuals with this are optimistic enough to put difficulties behind them and redirect their attention to positive means of coping. This is not easy to achieve however.

Consider the case study below and think about how you might help Melanie, a second year student, overcome the ongoing negative feelings she has about the following event.

Case Study 7.2

'I was asked by a health care assistant to help her with one of the patients, a large lady who required a hoist in order to be moved or handled. The health care assistant asked me to help her lift this patient onto the commode without any lifting aids or equipment. Having assessed the situation I knew it was unsafe to lift and so refused to do so without the use of a hoist. Having explained my reasons for not helping, I stated that if she got the appropriate equipment I would certainly assist her.

At first I felt proud that I had been assertive and that I had used my skills of assessment, making a decision relevant to the safety of the three of us. However, the health care assistant showed her disapproval in front of the patient and other members of staff. After that, I felt she took every opportunity to find fault with me and put me down. I know I made the right decision regarding patient harm and back injuries, but I still feel upset that I had been made to feel an "unpopular nurse" and in situations like this when I know I'm doing the right thing but others only want to get the job done quickly really get me down and make me feel like giving it all up.'

Compare your considerations with ours

First of all Melanie would need someone to listen emphathetically to what she was saying. You might have identified that it would be important to let her know that you understand and empathise with her by showing acceptance of her feelings, using the skills of paraphrasing, reflecting back and helping her to clarify her concerns and problems. It would be important to acknowledge feelings such as anger and wanting to give up her career.

To help her overcome her distress, we expect you have noted how important it would be to help Melanie to reflect on the positive aspects of the situation, about her caring skills, risk management, and her concern for the physical safety of her colleagues as well as the patient. Another positive aspect would have been recognition of the assertiveness skills she displayed and that she was acting in accordance with the NMC Code (2008). All this will reinforce that she is working well and that she should not 'lose heart' because of this one situation.

The question Melanie might find useful now is to consider what her next actions might be. When not so angry she might feel able to talk things over with the health care assistant, or she may need the assistance of her mentor or her personal tutor.

If you look back at the above you can see that Melanie might have used two types of coping strategies which have been identified in the literature: problem-focused and emotion-focused (Kozier *et al.*, 2008). Problem-focused coping strategies help by undertaking action which could improve a situation (in this case discussion about why it was so important to move a patient safely). However, Melanie also needed to find ways of relieving her emotional distress by using an emotion-focused strategy (in her case by using a reflective approach which would help her to get things into perspective and reinforce the value of the care she provided).

To think about

Have you ever been in a situation when you have been upset by what a colleague has said to you?

+ How well did you think you managed your feelings, or in other words, what coping strategies were you able to use?
+ What resources did you use to help you cope, e.g. people (colleagues, mentors, personal tutor, friend) or actions related to distraction or relaxation (e.g. physical exercise, meditation, yoga, reading, having a long bath). Try to be honest about any negative coping strategies you might use such as overuse of alcohol, taking your frustrations out on someone else, e.g. a family member or the cat.
+ What do you need to do in the future to remind yourself of your strengths and to cope with any prolonged negativity such as bearing a grudge?

The solution-focused approach (brief therapy or appreciative approach)

Various approaches have been used to try to get people to consider how to overcome difficulties. Miller and Berg (1995) describe the use of a solution-focused approach in their work, particularly with clients who have a history of alcohol abuse. They make the point that it is not unusual for an individual's strengths to be hidden beneath a mound of negative feelings, such as shame, guilt or disgust. They say that pain is a useful starting point for awareness and reflection but it does not help the solution. 'Pain may get us started, but strengths and resources help us to stay on track and finish the job' (Miller and Berg, 1995: 25). It is also evident that many of our patients experience this and may use inappropriate coping strategies. Niall, a student nurse, told us of the frustration he felt in caring for Tyrone, who experienced auditory hallucinations and delusions. Tyrone, frightened by these, found that the only way he felt he could cope was by getting very angry and shouting at the voices until they went away but also by engaging in alcohol and drug abuse. Changing these ineffective and damaging coping strategies was problematic and required a multi-professional approach, using appropriate resources, in order to help Tyrone to master his problems.

This strategy of focusing on solutions rather than only on problems has been useful in helping many people overcome difficulties by providing a more positive and constructive framework. For example in Alcoholics Anonymous people are asked to focus on the good parts of the day.

Getting, receiving and reflecting on feedback from others, helps us to become more aware of our strengths and resources which can then be used to our advantage in overcoming future problematic situations and combating adverse conditions. Consider how this might work in practice.

Case Study 7.3

'Lara was in her final clinical placement, an acute admissions unit, preparing for registration as a qualified staff nurse. She was feeling overwhelmed and asked to see Joanne, her personal guidance tutor. Joanne went to the unit and was concerned to see a tearful and distraught Lara. That day, although the unit was very busy, a decision had been made that Lara should lead a team so that she could work towards the proficiencies she needed in leadership and management skills. Lara said, "I hope to get a job on this unit when I qualify and the interviews will be coming up soon. I was here before as a second year student and I loved it so much so I asked to return for my final placement but this morning has been an absolute nightmare."

Joanne arranged to take her to a quiet place so they would have time to talk through the situation. Lara said, "I feel I have totally lost my confidence. I'll never be ready in time. How can I be a caring nurse and cope with all of this? I haven't even got the confidence to delegate any more. I feel as if I don't know what I'm doing."

Joanne listened to Lara's description of a whole series of events that had taken place that morning. Anxious relatives who had been concerned that their father wasn't receiving adequate care, pressure on beds resulting in a rapid turnover of admissions and transfers, junior staff who questioned the way she was delegating responsibilities, and a remark from another member of staff indicating that she would have to work faster if she was to be any use as a staff nurse. Joanne reminded herself that up to now she had not been aware of any problems with Lara's performance. On the contrary, she had received very positive comments from mentors throughout the programme and had always seemed to fit in well with colleagues.'

Joanne decided to use a solution-focused approach (adapted from McKergow and Clarke, 2005, with permission) to try to assist Lara to get back on track. In this a number of questions are used are used to help her move forward.

Think about a 'miracle'

Joanne asked Lara the following question: 'If you were to wake up tomorrow morning and a miracle had happened whilst you've been asleep and all your problems have gone, what would be the first thing that would be different and who would notice it?'

Lara started to describe herself as a perfect staff nurse who could cope with 'anything that was thrown at her'. She would be a nurse who was very calm, skilled and compassionate, very efficient and quick when undertaking tasks and highly regarded by everyone. Because Joanne wanted Lara to be able to describe this 'miracle' in as much detail as possible, they also looked at the NMC proficiencies and the job description for a junior qualified member of nursing staff. They made a note of what they would add to Lara's initial response to help to describe some of the professionally identified skills needed to reach the 'miracle'.

Lara thought that the first thing that she and then other people would notice would be that 'I would be more together'. Joanne asked her what this 'togetherness' would look like and Lara indicated that she would be calm in the chaos of everyday care and crisis situations and know what things to tackle first. Staff would listen to her and respond without too much moaning and groaning when she delegated. She would then be able to go off duty and relax without worrying all the time about what had happened that day.

Using a scaling question

Joanne then asked Lara to imagine a scale of 0 to 10, with the 'miracle' ranked as a 10 and 0 indicating no understanding or skills about what her image of a qualified nurse should do and be. She asked Lara to consider where she now placed herself on the scale. Lara thought she was at a 5 on the scale.

What has worked in the past and what resources were useful?

Joanne asked Lara to consider how she had reached that point on the scale, considering what strengths, achievements and resources she used. She assisted Lara in identifying what these were. She asked Lara to consider exceptions to the problems; situations when she hadn't panicked but felt in control, even if the unit was very busy. Lara described several situations when emergencies had happened and she felt she had responded well, although she hadn't been in overall charge.

Together they concluded that Lara had a variety of effective skills and resources that she could draw on and develop. For example, Lara had demonstrated that she was patient-focused in her care, was very methodical and responsive to acute situations, was highly motivated and had good time management skills. She wasn't frightened to ask questions and used a range of resources to enhance her learning including observation of good role models, used her reflective skills and written resources such as research articles and policies. Lara noted that in the past she was able to act as if she was calm even though she may have felt quite anxious inside. 'I've watched other people who seem calm,' she said, 'and I've tried to copy them.'

Taking small steps forward

Joanne asked Lara what she could do now to reach a 5.5 or a 6 on the scale. This was achieved by, firstly, looking at her 'miracle' and also reminding herself again of the internal and external resources available to her. In other words, what she had found to work well in the past and why. Joanne then asked Lara to identify something that she could achieve by the following week which was observable, achievable, realistic, specific and measurable. Lara said that she would try not to show how panicky she felt inside; instead she would act in a calm manner. She would do this by continuing to work towards the leadership and management proficiencies (related to delegating tasks) but take particular notice of when she was successful in maintaining a calm manner and when she was unable to do this and why. She would ask her mentor to give her specific feedback.

Lara also remembered that one of her resources in the past had been the keeping of a personal reflective diary. She thought this was a good way of monitoring her progress if she was honest and documented when she felt calm and self-assured as well as situations where she might have displayed lack of confidence and anxiety. She then needed to analyse her thoughts, feelings and behaviour and learn from her successes. Joanne then reminded her that key to her progress would be to do more of what works well, e.g. she might try giving a rationale to staff of why she had delegated in a particular way. If she found that this approach was time-consuming and led to arguments, she could leave this unsuccessful method and try a different approach.

Moving on up the scale

Lara and Joanne discussed the rationale for, and the implications of, continuing the solution-focused approach with Lara's mentor who agreed to help. Her mentor pointed out that Lara wouldn't have to get to a 10 by the end of the placement - perhaps 8 or 9 would be more realistic. Nobody was expecting that kind of miracle!

The mentor felt that one of the problems for Lara was that she had had too great an expectation of herself in too short a time and that the solution-focused approach would really help her by breaking down her ultimate target into achievable goals and would help her to appreciate and use her successes along the way.

For Lara this approach was very successful and helped her to gain all of her proficiencies by the end of the placement. In addition, she was enthusiastic about the way this had helped her to prepare for a successful job interview because she had looked so carefully at her detailed 'miracle' image of a staff nurse and her own strengths and resources. She knew what was expected of a qualified nurse and had the confidence and self-esteem to perform well at interview.

Application of the solution-focused approach to patient care

McAllister (2003) sees the solution orientation of this approach as an exciting way forward for nursing in terms of both professional development and care for clients. Whilst the part that problem-solving can play is acknowledged, focusing on what is going right and building on strengths, achievements and capacity can help maximise potential. She explains that during periods of stress, thinking becomes more rigid. As Lara found, it is hard to look beyond the problem. McAllister questions whether the problem-based approach alone, useful though it might be in many ways, is tending to constrain nursing and may also have a negative effect on the client in terms of the balance of power. 'Being the problem-solver works to privilege and illuminate the health carer's actions, whilst the work of being a client, struggling to survive, overcome and maintain resilience is overlooked' (McAllister, 2003: 530). The solution-focused approach, with its orientation towards the identification and use of personal strengths, qualities and resources, is therefore well suited to nursing and may help us to articulate the importance of and develop effective, caring approaches in partnership with patients and their families.

To think about

Think of a goal which you would like to achieve over the next few months. Follow the steps in the framework used by Joanne to help Lara to see if a solution-based approach might help you in your development.

+ Ask yourself the 'miracle' question - describe the 'perfect' state you would like to be in.
+ Say where you are now on an imaginary scale from 0 to 10, with the 'miracle' ranked as 10.
+ Write down what strengths, achievements and resources you have used to reach the point where you are now on the scale.
+ Think about what small steps you could take to reach the next point up on the scale. Remind yourself again of the internal and external resources available to you. Think carefully about how you will be able to tell that you have achieved it - in other words set yourself a realistic and observable goal.
+ Move up the scale by continuing to take a series of small steps. Do more of what works well and if something is not working try something different. You might want to consider at what point you will be satisfied that you have reached your maximum point on the scale taking into account the stage in your professional development. It might take some time to reach 'perfection' depending on the nature of the goal you set yourself. However, the scaling approach will help you to clarify the direction you need to take and to feel good about the distance you have travelled. It will also help you to remember your strengths and the resources you can use.

How building up our emotional resilience will help us to care

You will remember from Lara's story that her initial lack of confidence led to her feeling inadequate, overwhelmed and therefore not able to think clearly and function as effectively as she might. Using the solution-focused approach to help her identify her strengths, being more aware of her successes and the resources available began to make her think and feel very differently about herself. In other words she became more emotionally resilient in that she would be more likely in the future to perceive challenges or problems as learning opportunities. According to Tusaie and Dyer (2004: 3), resilience is 'a combination of abilities and characteristics that interact dynamically and allow an individual to bounce back, cope successfully and function above the norm in spite of significant stress or adversity.'

As we have found, the management of our emotions has important implications for practice since memory functions best when the mind is calm, influencing our capacity to pay attention and pick up cues (Abraham, 2004). Nurses often refer to the way in which they 'cope' with situations and earlier we described problem-focused and emotion-focused strategies. Using strategies such a the solution-focused approach will help support and develop an individual's strengths and therefore their ability to cope with difficult, new or challenging situations. Coping and resilience are related concepts but coping refers to the thinking and behaviour we use to manage the demands of specific stressful situations whereas resilience refers to an overall or more generalised ability (Campbell-Sills et al., 2006).

An increase in self-awareness can help us to make a more rational judgement of our capabilities and reactions and, if we feel any criticism unjustified, to seek constructive dialogue (Abraham, 2004). We need therefore to learn to apply the same kind of critical analysis to ourselves as we apply to our academic work. Becoming more aware and analytical about our emotional reactions to situations will help us not only to regain equilibrium but also to recognise inappropriate or unhelpful reactions. Jackson et al. (2007: 6), however, suggest that nurses need help to do this, by focusing on ways in which personal resilience can be fostered. They identify five main ways for facilitating this: building positive nurturing relationships and networks, maintaining positivity, developing emotional insight, achieving life balance and spirituality, and becoming more reflective.

We can therefore enhance our resilience by engaging in reflective practice and utilising strategies which help us to develop our strengths and focus on solutions to things we find difficult. We can also be helped by receiving positive feedback and encouragement, perhaps through clinical supervision, mentor and peer group support, building up a network of people who 'nurture' us by giving us support and guidance (which will help us to maintain our motivation and positivity). However, we also have to ensure that we give ourselves time to renew ourselves, achieving what Jackson et al. (2007) call a 'life balance'. We can do this by various methods of relaxation and stress reduction but also by making time for other priorities in our lives such as family and friends. Finding the best balance between work, study, family and social life is sometimes difficult but this is essential if we are to function effectively. The more resilient we are, the more effective we will be as caring nurses.

We should also be aware of the importance of helping to develop resilience in others, including colleagues and patients. This will be particularly important following registration when you will move into a leadership and management role and also in your ongoing interactions with families and carers. Helping others to become more resilient can be achieved through engaging in support and encouragement but also by working in partnership with them to identify and use the internal and external resources available to them, as we saw in Chapter 5.

Caring is using our creativity to find solutions

In the complex and often highly organised world of professional care we may forget how our personal experiences and knowledge may be an important resource. Read the following published story in which Perry (2005: 45) describes how she used a creative approach and drew on her own memories as a resource to help calm an extremely restless and agitated 85-year-old man.

Case Study 7.4

'Then I heard him repeat a series of words in a garbled fashion and recognised the words of an old hymn. I began to sing the hymn and immediately he became quiet. The change was instantaneous and profound. … As long as the hymns were sung the patient rested. … I loved being his nurse because none of the textbook interventions worked. He required flexible, creative nurses who were not afraid to try the unconventional and who were willing to stay. Large doses of sedation made no difference. Somewhere in the deepest levels of this man's mind our presence through music and just being near him touched him. It was a profound night because all my years of training and education came down to the simple singing of a song and using music to touch his soul.'

For us, the account highlights the artistry of caring. Artists are creative and have the ability to look at things in a different way – they help us to see things in a new light. Perry (2005) noticed the familiar words of a hymn and then used her knowledge of this to find a creative way of communicating with the patient. It is sometimes in everyday ways that we can use our creativity. One of our students recalled a situation which occurred during a visit to a client in the community. He needed his feet soaking but the only bowl available was a washing-up bowl. The qualified nurse decided to leave the foot care for another time but was impressed when the student suggested using a plastic bag to line the bowl so that the care could be implemented there and then. The client was very grateful as, because of the student's creative approach, he was given immediate relief from his discomfort.

To think about

Reflect on the ways in which nurse–patient relationships can become therapeutic and healing by using our creativity.

+ Think of ways in which this occurs in everyday practice – perhaps through humour, shared interests, appropriate self-disclosure, conversations, play, touch and actions.
+ Think of situations which you have seen or perhaps experienced yourself in which 'unusual' caring approaches were used to benefit the patient. They could include, for example, the use of art, poetry, play, music, drama.
+ Do you think we recognise and use and value ourselves as a valuable therapeutic and creative resource?

The artistry of caring can be seen within nurse-patient relationships. McAllister (2003: 533) claims that nursing needs to remind itself and others of its uniqueness as a profession because 'it has as its essence the human qualities of nurturance, care, presence and connection.' Work by Dame Cicely Saunders (2002: 30), founder of the hospice movement in the UK, reinforces this. She says that it is the very way care is given that can 'reach the most hidden places and that this may be an enabler of a search for spiritual peace.' She describes a male patient with incontinence being reassured by being told that 'it's the disease not you.' The patient describes how he gradually came to forget 'that silly male pride' because the nurses talked to him all the time they were washing and changing him, undertaking the task with such dignity and care that in the end he said he found that 'he didn't give a damn'. In other words, the nurses transformed a situation which could have been undignified and embarrassing for him (affecting his self-image and self-esteem) into one of acceptance and self-respect.

This is an example of the importance of the artistry of care. When this artistry is missing, it can lead to negative emotions such as distress and loss of hope as seen in Chapter 3, and can detrimentally affect health or the journey to a peaceful death. By articulating and reflecting on the way we give care, we can see the importance of the care we have given. We can use it as a way of reinforcing the value of the relationships we develop with our patients and clients. It is easy to overlook these aspects as important successes, all of which could add to the way in which we are able to see ourselves in a positive light and value what we bring of ourselves to our profession. The more we articulate these aspects, the more we are likely to value ourselves and others will value us too.

Helping patients to draw on and develop their own resources

As we have said, it is often when undertaking perhaps the simplest tasks of nursing that we are able to touch another human being deeply as they struggle for meaning and hope in their life.

Case Study 7.5

'Tom was recovering from an amputation of his right leg. He was very quiet and didn't seem to want to make conversation. He rarely asked for help and, as he was MRSA positive, was isolated in a single room and didn't see many people. I thought that being alone and immobile was what was bothering him. One day, I was helping him to shower and dress (a time-consuming process) when I managed to engage him in conversation. He talked about holidays he had enjoyed in the past but said that now because of his amputation he wouldn't be able to plan another. I didn't feel I could reassure him that holidays were possible because I didn't want to give him false hopes about goals he might not be able to achieve.

When the dressing came off he asked me what the wound was like. I asked him if he would like to see the scar. He refused at first but I offered him a mirror and said that if he couldn't look at it at that time I could take the mirror away again. He then said he wanted to see it and so I placed the mirror in front of him. He sort of yelled at first but I just sat quietly and asked if he wanted the mirror taken away. He didn't. He looked a while longer and then said that it didn't look that bad now that he had seen it. He spoke about a friend of his who had had an amputation during the war in a prisoner-of-war camp without anaesthetic using a meat knife and a saw. He said that if his friend could still go on holiday with one leg then so could he.

He seemed a lot better, and when his wife visited him he asked for a haircut. I couldn't believe the change in his appearance. He looked younger, his eyes were twinkling and he was smiling. He admitted to being quite vain for a 'man of his age' and was more worried about how his amputation appeared to people. I was quite wrong to think that he was worried about his mobility. I think that because he was elderly I missed the fact that his appearance would still be very important. I won't forget that lesson.'

This account is important because it reminds us of what we mean by caring. The student helped Tom to draw on his own resources, through her interactions, and helped him to articulate them and reframe his problem. He overcame his fear of the scar and in doing so he was able to make comparisons with his friend's experience and gain a renewed sense of hope and dignity. As a nurse you will be sharing precious and important moments with others as they struggle to come to terms with perhaps a long-term or stressful condition, loss, altered body image or even death. Many nurses see the fact that they are able to get so close to others in moments of extreme sadness but also moments of extreme happiness as a great privilege which can be regarded as a spiritual dimension of nursing. Watson (1988) describes this kind of close interaction which takes place between patient and nurse as transpersonal – a spiritual union – one in which deep experience is shared.

Spirituality as a resource in health care

People who belong to a particular faith may be helped to understand and make sense of their lives, and consideration of an individual's religious needs is an important aspect of holistic assessment, whatever their age. Gaining knowledge of or information about resources we can use to help people to practise and gain solace from their faith is an important part of a nurse's role. However, we may fail to help many patients if we think only in terms of organised religion. Moss (2002: 40) quotes Buber (1957), a Jewish theologian, who once observed that there is nothing like religion 'for hiding the face of God' and highlights the fact that practitioners in health and social care are often faced with clients who are searching for meaning in their lives, a significant spiritual quest. You may have come across patients who have asked you the question 'Why me?' or have shown signs of despair or loss of hope or purpose. We may feel that responding to spiritual concerns like this is not part of our role but Moss (2002: 44) reminds us that 'We can no more give a sense of meaning and purpose to someone else than we can eat or breathe for them. But to share that journey with them can help them feel valued; which is the first step to a regaining of purpose and meaning.'

Wright (2006) also suggests that meaning, value and hope signify a great deal to people but may be relegated down the list of priorities behind organisational and clinical matters. We can only do this by valuing ourselves and also our colleagues. He discusses work in Scotland where students of nursing, divinity and medicine come together to explore spirituality and health in their work with people with mental health problems and learning disabilities. 'Our aim is to help professionals develop more whole, more compassionate, more spiritual approaches to care that are integrated into everyday work. But we can only talk seriously about this when we have successfully made this a multidisciplinary approach' (Wright, 2006: 25). The author claims that as people learn to experience and understand patients differently so their practice begins to change. Learning together across disciplines is a valuable method of building up team resources and acknowledging the contribution each profession can make.

Summary

In this chapter we have discussed that, as a student, you experience all kinds of demanding situations and pressures which can lead to excessive stress. We have highlighted the importance of recognising and managing this and of looking after yourself. If you see the relevance and value of the work you are undertaking and have the ability to 'bounce back' when meeting challenges or adversity, you will be less likely to be at risk of becoming overwhelmed and experience emotional exhaustion. Your emotional resilience will develop if you are able to see solutions as well as problems or difficulties and acknowledge and use the strengths and resources of yourself and others. Some of our strengths and resources may be overlooked, such as our creativity and the close and 'spiritual' relationships we develop with patients and clients. These all help us to improve our 'artistry' in caring and also help to sustain positive feelings about ourselves.

We have also suggested that a solution-focused approach is a beneficial tool both for our own development and also for use in the development of others including patients/clients and their families. You may have noticed strong parallels between this chapter and Chapter 5 (Working in partnerships with carers) because many of the caring indicators useful for helping us as professionals to care for ourselves also help us to care for others and to recognise their needs within the caring process (e.g. through the giving and receiving of positive feedback, feeling valued, knowing and using a range of resources and coping with competing demands). This underlines the importance of understanding more about the nature of caring and valuing caring as the central aspect of nursing as we share with others in our common humanity.

Looking forward

In Chapter 8, we will revisit and integrate the caring indicators which we have uncovered and specified at the end of each chapter. This resource will provide us with an overview of the 'artistry' of a caring nurse.

Activity

Think about personal aspects which you might have but want to develop further. The following framework will help you to take responsibility for your personal and professional development. You may find it useful to write down your answers to the questions which are loosely based on Goleman's (1999: 26) personal competency framework. Your answers could form the basis of a personal action plan or a dialogue with your mentor or a trusted critical friend.

Are you self-aware?

+ Give an example of your ability to recognise your emotions and their effects on your performance.
+ Make a list of your strengths and areas for further development.
+ How do feel about yourself in terms of your self-worth and capabilities?

How do you self-regulate – manage your emotions, impulses and resources?

+ Describe a time when you were able to keep disruptive emotions and impulses in check and/or a time you found it difficult.
+ Give an example of a time you've been honest or conscientious in your practice e.g. admitted a lack of knowledge or skill, truth telling, demonstrated how well you can work with other team members.
+ Give an example of how you have been flexible and/or innovative in your approach to practice.

Are you motivated?

+ Describe ways in which you have improved or worked towards achieving a standard of excellence.
+ Give an example of the way you made use of a learning opportunity the last time you were in practice.
+ How persistent have you been in pursuing goals despite obstacles and setbacks?

Please don't be too hard on yourself but use this as a guide for honest self-development.

Caring indicators

1. Recognising times of particular stress for individuals and groups, e.g. during life transitions and periods of loss and change
2. Finding ways of caring for ourselves in order to care for others
3. Acknowledging and using our own internal and external strengths and resources and helping patients, relatives and colleagues to do the same
4. Recognising the impact of negative coping strategies on self and the care we provide
5. Developing positive coping strategies to deal with stress, e.g. time for renewal
6. Being aware of and avoiding 'stress contagion' and negativity
7. Recognising indicators of burnout in health care professionals and the effects it can have on patient care
8. Becoming more aware of and analytical about our emotional reactions to situations
9. Moving from problems to solutions
10. Caring for ourselves by developing emotional resilience
11. Helping colleagues, patients and carers to develop resilience
12. Caring by drawing on personal resources such as our creativity and innovative thinking
13. Caring as a spiritual union in which deep experience is shared
14. Helping others in their search for meaning and hope
15. Recognising how others can gain comfort and hope through religious beliefs and needs
16. Promoting a culture in which team members feel valued and have a shared sense of purpose

References

Abraham, R (2004) Emotional competence as antecedent to performance: a contingency framework. *Genetic, Social and General Psychology Monographs* **130**, 117-143.

Campbell-Sills, L, Cohan, S and Stein, M (2006) Relationship of resilience to personality, coping and psychiatric symptoms in young adults. *Behaviour Research and Therapy* **44**, 585-599.

Covey, S (1999) *The Seven Habits of Highly Effective People.* London: Simon & Schuster.

Edward, K and Hercelinskyj, G (2007) Burnout in the caring nurse: learning resilient behaviours. *British Journal of Nursing* **16**, 240-242.

Glasberg, A, and Eriksson, S Norberg, A (2007) Burnout and 'stress of conscience' among health care personnel. *Journal of Advanced Nursing* **57**, 392-403.

Goleman, D (1999) *Working with Emotional intelligence.* London: Bloomsbury.

Jackson, D, Firtko, A and Edenborough, M (2007) Personal resilience as a strategy for surviving and thriving in the face of workplace adversity: a literature review. *Journal of Advanced Nursing* **60**, 1, 1-9.

Kozier, B, Erb, G, Berman, A, Snyder, S, Lake, R and Harvey, S (2008) *Fundamentals of Nursing: Concepts, process and practice.* Harlow: Pearson Education.

McAllister, M (2003) Doing practice differently: solution-focused nursing. *Journal of Advanced Nursing* **41**, 528-535.

McKergow, M and Clarke, J (2005) *Positive Approaches to Change: Applications of Solutions Focus and Appreciative Inquiry at Work.* Cheltenham: Solutions Books.

Miller, S and Berg, I (1995) *The Miracle Method: A radically new approach to problem drinking.* London: Norton & Company.

Moss, B (2002) Spirituality: a personal view. In Thompson, N (ed) *Loss and Grief.* Basingstoke: Palgrave.

NMC (Nursing and Midwifery Council) (2008) *The Code: Standards of conduct, performance and ethics for nurses and midwives.* London: Nursing and Midwifery Council.

Perry, B (2005) Core nursing values brought to life through stories. *Nurisng standard,* **7**, 41-48.

Saunders, C (2002) *The Philosophy of Hospice.* In Thompson, N (ed) *Loss and Grief.* Basingstoke: Palgrave.

Smith, A (2003) Learning about reflection. PhD thesis, University of Northumbria, Newcastle upon Tyne.

Tusaie, K and Dyer, J (2004) Resilience: a historical review of the construct. *Holistic Nursing Practice* **18**, 3-8.

Watson, J (1988) *Nursing: Human science and human care. A theory of nursing.* New York: National League for Nursing.

Wicks, R (2006) *Overcoming Secondary Stress in Medical and Nursing Practice.* New York: Oxford University Press.

Wilkes, G (2002) Introduction: a second generation of resilience research. *Journal of Clinical Psychology* **58**, 229-232.

Wright, S (2006) Spirited approach. *Nursing Standard* **20**, 24-25.

Chapter 8
Reviewing the caring indicators

LEARNING OBJECTIVES

By the end of this chapter you should have an understanding of:

1. A new overview of the caring indicators which were summarised at the end of previous chapters
2. Aspects of caring which we have categorised in the themes of: Being and Becoming, Overcoming Obstacles, Noticing and Doing
3. An initial framework from which you can further develop your understanding of the nature of caring and of ways in which you can enhance your caring skills

Introduction

The indicators highlighted at the end of each chapter, which emerged as a result of our discussions, helped us to focus on the nature of caring. We brought the indicators all together and then found that we could categorise them into four key themes:

1. Being and becoming
2. Overcoming obstacles
3. Noticing
4. Doing

Caring is about connecting to others and we found that the initial letters of these four themes reflected this important aspect by forming the apt word BOND. In this chapter we have outlined the main characteristics emerging which describe each of the four themes. We hope this framework will assist you in the process of understanding, appreciating and articulating caring which is at the heart of effective nursing practice.

Using the BOND framework

Before you look at the framework (Table 8.1) in detail, consider the following scenario which occurred when we were undertaking a group tutorial with a number of nursing students after they had completed a practice placement.

Case Study 8.1

The students commented that they felt they were 'drowning' in the heavy workload and were feeling emotionally drained and worn out. They said they were glad to be back in the university as it gave them a break from the emotional and physical demands of placement. They started talking about guilt feelings, saying they believed they had sometimes not responded enough to patient needs. They also shared examples of how they had been affected emotionally, for example when caring for dying and very ill patients and also when they had to help distressed relatives and in empathising with them, they identified with their experiences. After becoming upset following a particularly harrowing episode, Paula, one of the students, commented that she had been told by a staff nurse that 'nurses have to be hard' and Paula was 'too soft and too caring'.

To think about

+ Consider the incident described above. What aspects do Paula and the other students need to think about in order to understand how being caring has consequences for the nurse in terms of emotional stability and how can nurses manage this? Do they need to be hard to survive?
+ You might want to use bits of the BOND framework (Table 8.1) outlined on page 137, to help with your reflections and also you might want to draw on pertinent literature to help with a deeper analysis.

Compare your considerations with those of our students

We found the BOND framework gave us pointers to help in our reflective discussion with the students. When Paula first said that she had been told that 'nurses have to be hard' a number of the other students agreed with this to some extent. We asked them to look at the BOND framework and consider the 'being' theme. All agreed that these were characteristics that they did not want to lose but more importantly wanted to keep and develop. They then moved on to the next theme and identified that 'being hard' could be an obstacle which had to be managed or overcome. However, they had also noticed ('noticing' is the third theme of the framework) that they had become emotionally and physically drained. They suggested that they could use these feelings as an incentive for understanding better why this had occurred. They recognised that it was important to move on to the final theme of the framework of doing something positive to manage their feelings. Considering the 'caring by doing' theme helped them to see that they had not been caring for themselves adequately, for example by having too high expectations of themselves and also having unrealistic feelings that they had to make everyone feel better. One student commented that the framework themes were all inter-related in that you needed to notice what you were doing, be conscientious about uncovering and 'dealing with obstacles' (the second theme), be a caring person to yourself as well as for others in order to be what you wanted to be. We all thought this comment, although rather convoluted, helped us understand some of the complexity and 'work' needed in order to be and become a caring nurse.

We helped the students to go on further with their critical analysis by using imagery and metaphor to think again about what it meant to be 'hard'. They decided that something which is hard, although it might be tough, could also be inflexible and brittle and so would be likely to break under pressure. They thought that people who were hard were often insensitive, unkind, forceful, and sometimes self-centred and ruthless.

Some nurses appeared 'hard' when they distanced themselves from others and became task oriented rather than person-centred, probably to avoid feeling vulnerable and getting hurt. The students said they hoped that they wouldn't be like that even when they had more responsibilities in the future. They discussed whether this hardness might be a sign of 'professional burnout' and possibly could be the end result of being too 'soft' and overwhelmed with emotions. This process would have an adverse effect on the individual nurse and would also affect their ability to help patients, relatives and colleagues as much as they should. One student commented that she had read somewhere that nurses have to have a degree of 'hardiness' rather than being hard. The other students liked this description as it helped them to reframe the issue, conjuring up a different image - one in which the nurse could still be emotionally and therapeutically connected but tough enough to acknowledge his or her limitations and be able to 'bounce back' when feeling under pressure and overwhelmed.

They concluded that the framework itself had helped them to understand that in order to stay caring they could use their emotional responses, understand them and learn different ways of managing them. We advised them to look for academic literature in order to understand more about the nature of emotional intelligence, particularly in its relationship with personal resilience. We provided them with Tusaie and Dyer's (2004: 3) definition of emotional resilience which we used in Chapter 7, 'a combination of abilities and characteristics that interact dynamically and allow an individual to bounce back, cope successfully and function above the norm in spite of significant stress or adversity.' We also discussed work by Abraham (2004) who indicated that memory functions best when the mind is calm, influencing our capacity to pay attention and pick up cues.

The students commented that they could more easily look back calmly and critically reflect when they were away from the situation. Although they acknowledged that reflection is part of good practice, in the rush and bustle of everyday working life it is often easier to reflect more systematically and get things into 'better proportion' when away from the situation. One student suggested that keeping a personal diary helped her to do this.

Table 8.1 BOND - A framework for reflecting on the nature of caring

B Caring by being and becoming	O Caring by overcoming obstacles	N Caring by noticing	D Caring by doing
+ Being a caring presence	+ Developing resilience	+ Increasing our sensitivity and learning more about the skills of noticing	+ Preparing the ground for, and maintaining, caring relationships
+ Being empathetic in order to 'tune into' and help others	+ Reframing the problem or issue	+ Noticing the effects of cues and interactions on ourselves	+ Understanding and supporting informal carers
+ Becoming more emotionally intelligent and competent	+ Using preventative and restorative skills	+ Noticing indicators of burnout and the effects stress can have on patient care	+ Engaging in critical analysis of practice
+ Being conscientious	+ Making caring in teams effective		+ Caring for yourself and influencing the working environment
+ Being adaptable, flexible and creative			

Time to think back

Did you find you could relate to the experiences of our students? You may have found your considerations took you down a similar path to ours, but don't worry if you took a different stance. You may have extended your knowledge by undertaking a literature search, perhaps by using key words such as 'stress/stress management', 'emotional intelligence', 'hardiness', 'emotional resilience', 'emotional labour', 'burnout'. The articles we have found particularly useful related to hardiness and emotional resilience are by Jacelon (1997) and Jackson et al. (2007) and concerning emotional intelligence in nursing work, the article by McQueen (2004) is interesting and pertinent. You will find the full references for these at the end of this chapter.

Looking again at the framework

We used an example of working with our students and using the BOND framework to help demonstrate to you its potential for understanding the complex nature of caring. As we noted in the learning outcomes at the beginning of this chapter, we wanted to provide you with an initial framework from which you could continue to develop your understanding of the nature of caring and of ways in which you could enhance your caring skills. We hope you will find opportunities to use the framework to discover more about caring throughout your future career, as this search for learning should be 'a never-ending journey'. The framework therefore is meant as a prompt for continuation of learning rather than a finished product. The simplicity of the framework is a strength but also a limitation. The intricacies of caring behaviour may not be immediately obvious. Therefore you will also find it useful to revisit the detail of the caring indicators which occur at the end of each chapter. We are sure you will find more dimensions and characteristics if you continue to unravel and analyse the complexity of caring. For the moment we will look back to give you a summary of the content within the themes of the BOND framework.

Caring by being and becoming

As we have seen throughout the book, caring is linked with what we are like as people. In nursing we learn 'to be and become' (perhaps you've noticed how much you have changed in order to perform your role) as well as learn about the knowledge and practice skills required. As a student you experience many different situations and challenges and these may lead to reappraisals of how you view yourself, both in the present and what you might become in the future. You may find you are changing in your perceptions, perhaps of others or about what you see as important in your life. Many of your hopes, fears and aspirations are likely to change over time.

From the stories outlined in the chapters in this book, we have seen the influences of individual nurses on the way care is experienced. Our beliefs, values and characteristics affect our identity and how we are perceived both as a person and as a professional. In nursing we attach a great deal of importance to the therapeutic use of 'self' and inherent within this is recognition of what we bring to situations and interactions with others in a positive sense. However, we have also seen ways in which we can affect others in a negative way. The theme of 'being and becoming' highlights the active search in which we need to engage in order to understand ourselves and develop awareness of what we are and how this influences how we act. If we understand ourselves we will be better able to understand and help others so that we can ensure we are caring in our approaches.

Being a caring presence

To demonstrate this we have seen that we must be ready to connect to and be available for patients, families and significant others. In doing so, we will be acknowledging our common humanity and ourselves and others as 'spiritual' beings. We will be able to see caring as a 'spiritual union' in which deep experience may be shared. This is a great privilege for us as nurses and is one which you may be interested in researching further in the future. To us, spirituality in nursing, regardless of whether or not we are religious, includes the opportunities to share with others in their search for meaning and hope. We have found that all our caring relationships are a two-way process. The stories also tell us that there is likely to be an exchange of emotional gifts and we need to be aware of and appreciate the benefits gained by us as carers as well as those being cared for. We need therefore to avoid falling into the trap of being professionally arrogant but recognise that as professionals we are part of a continuum of care often in partnership with informal carers.

Being empathetic in order to 'tune into' and help others

Empathy is different from sympathy which really just means feeling sorry for the other person. By being empathetic, we move our gaze (or focus and concentration) from the body (as an object of intervention) to the person (the individual living a life). We are able to connect to others through using our communication skills which may include the effective use of touch, humour and silence. We are also respectful to others, irrespective of their age, gender, cultural origins, class, status or condition from which they suffer. The stories indicated that the skills of empathy also include being alert to client 'readiness' for information or life changes.

Becoming more emotionally intelligent and competent

We have found that we need to become more aware of and analytical about ourselves - recognising and learning from our own emotions and their effects. Just like the students at the beginning of this chapter, we can increase our emotional awareness by learning from feelings such as anger, frustration, fears, guilt and sadness. We can manage our emotions, not by suppressing them, but by learning ways in which we can become more self-controlled, keeping disruptive or overwhelming emotions and impulses in check so that we can carry on with our work of helping others. This will increase our competency in coping with situations and therefore increase our self-confidence. We also found that individuals learn from factors which motivate and influence them such as hope and determination and it is also important to become more aware of and acknowledge our capabilities and resources. It is only too easy to dwell on our limitations rather than our strengths.

Becoming more emotionally intelligent enables us to become more caring by recognising the positive and negative effects of our emotional responses. For example we can understand the effects of significant incidents in practice such as in relationships in which immediate rapport is established (described as 'clicking') and also those which engender fears, prejudices and stereotyping within us.

Being conscientious

As we have seen in the stories, being conscientious often involves going the 'extra mile' and also being ready to take personal responsibility for our caring work. It means that we are prepared to engage in emotional as well as physical labour. By being conscientious, we will also be motivated and committed, compassionate, genuine, warm and sensitive.

Being adaptable, flexible and creative

We are able to become more caring by drawing on personal resources such as our creativity or innovative thinking and by making the most of opportunities to show we care. We can also develop our creativity and imagination in different ways by using a range of resources such as literature, art, poetry and music and by learning to think more metaphorically.

Caring by overcoming obstacles

We know that the very nature of nursing work means that we meet many problems and obstacles. These may be both personally derived (related to our thoughts, feelings, beliefs and attitudes) and situation derived (perhaps due to pressure and the nature of our workload, organisational constraints and influences, or team conflicts). From the stories which triggered our discussions, we have identified not only a number of obstacles which nurses have to overcome in order to be or remain caring but also a range of strategies which can assist us to do this. Taking problems home may have an adverse impact on our personal relationships and social life; and conversely we may also experience problematic and demanding life events which can impact on the way we act professionally.

Developing resilience

One of the ways in which we can develop our resilience so that we have more hardiness and ability to cope with workplace adversity and stress is to gain a positive self-concept. As we have seen, this can influence the ways in which we respond to others and also to challenging situations. We must learn to be aware of and value our strengths and capabilities. Reflecting on these will enable us to move from problems to solutions and learn ways of developing a range of positive coping strategies so that our self-confidence is enhanced. Another way of caring for ourselves and increasing our overall emotional resilience is utilising other strategies such as maintaining a balance between work and other aspects of our lives, engaging in relaxing and de-stressing activities, taking notice of helpful feedback, and building up 'nurturing' relationships perhaps with fellow students, mentors and other colleagues.

Reframing the problem or issue

We have found that sometimes in situations which engender within us an emotional response (e.g. fear, frustration, anger, disappointment, sadness) we are unable to think or act clearly or rationally. The stress becomes distress and blocks our ability to manage the situation effectively. One of the key ways of changing a distressing situation into a manageable one is to alter how we think about and perceive it. For example, changing perceptions that we have of limitations in our knowledge or skills into opportunities for learning is an example of reframing. In Chapter 7, we saw how a student was able to use her fears and anxieties about her perceived deficiencies as a useful starting point for her development. With help, she was able to reframe her problems using a solution-focused approach. At the beginning of this chapter we saw how a group of students reframed their approach to the problem of becoming 'hard' by using images and metaphors.

We found that when we care for others there may be barriers in communication which need to be recognised and overcome. Reframing issues and seeing people as people not as problems will be a first step in achieving this. There may also be occasions when we need to suspend our judgement of another's behaviour and lifestyle. We are always in danger of using our various professional or personal frameworks as explanations rather than listening enough to patients and their families. In doing so we may make assumptions and jump to hasty and even inappropriate conclusions. Caring therefore means being closely attentive to others and open-minded enough to consider alternative explanations and approaches - an ongoing process of reframing.

Using preventative and restorative skills

Proactive interventions and risk assessments are an essential part of the preventative caring process. However, in the rush and bustle of routines and procedures something obvious can easily be missed or assumptions can be made. With a focus on completing tasks in a limited amount of time, the 'person' may be lost and important opportunities for the nurturing and restorative/healing aspects of nursing care missed. As we found in Chapter 4, it may be quiet and compliant patients who may not gain the care they need because they were not asked. Not only does proactive care engender trust and feelings of being safe and cared for, but it also helps prevent problems occurring in the first place.

As we have seen, we may also 'lose' the person because of how we perceive them as problems particularly if they are hostile and aggressive. We can be helped by policies and organisational procedures such as those related to 'zero tolerance' and handling difficult situations. Perspectives and guidance can also be gained from academic knowledge and also through undertaking reflective activities. This will widen our understanding and increase our skills in preventing and managing such challenges. We know from our discussions how important it is for any individual to feel cared for even if they show behaviour which is challenging or problematic for us. If anyone does not feel cared for, this can have a negative impact on his or her self-image and their ability to cope with illness, anxieties or adversity. In working with patients and their families, we need to understand that there are times of particular stress which may occur perhaps during life transitions or periods of frustration, loss and change. We can work in partnership with patients, relatives and colleagues to help them to find and use their strengths and resources to overcome difficulties or adjust to new challenges.

Making caring in teams effective

We have to overcome obstacles to our ability to be caring which may sometimes be related to organisational pressures and demands from wider socio-political and economic factors. Because of the inevitable rapidly changing world of health and social care, it is important that individual members of a health and social care teams value each other and the particular contribution each can make. We need to find ways of articulating to others the importance of the caring work we as nurses undertake so it may gain the recognition it deserves. However, although we have tended to focus on the individual in this book, we can only achieve so much on our own. We can overcome obstacles and achieve much more if we are members of a cohesive and collaborative team. It is even more important given the changing nature of care provision for the team to work in partnership with patients and their families. We need all the knowledge and skills of the multidisciplinary team but also of relatives and carers so they can be used for the good of the patient or client.

Caring by noticing

The caring indicators have shown us the importance of 'noticing' - picking up cues which may be otherwise not apparent or hidden. This sensitivity to others is at the centre of our ability to communicate effectively and show empathy and compassion. We have to use our senses (seeing, hearing, smelling and touching) to notice, and also our interpretations and feelings about people and situations, which may be almost 'unconscious' (sometimes known as intuition). However, sometimes we may not 'notice', perhaps deliberately as a defence mechanism, to prevent us getting involved or because we are focusing on tasks which have to be achieved in a very short time. It is therefore useful to look again at the indicators to see how noticing is integral to caring.

Increasing our sensitivity and learning more about the skills of noticing

Noticing is a key skill in nursing. Nurses engage in complex observations and interactions and need to be particularly sensitive if they are to be able to pick up not only the obvious but also the more subtle or hidden cues, which may be physical, emotional, spiritual, educational or social in origin. The stories have also indicated that effective nurses are able to notice when there are opportunities for establishing connectedness in relationships with patients and others. For example they use skills in being able to recognise when a client and their family are in a state of 'readiness' for supportive help, information and health education. They are also sensitive to religious and cultural needs and preferences and are proactive by asking patients what they need. They also make every effort to notice the effects of their interactions in order to develop optimum emotional and physical health in others.

We can use a variety of reflective activities in order to learn more about the art of noticing. In doing so, we can increase our sensitivity and awareness. We will widen and enhance our caring skills if we also use our observation skills to notice and learn from the ways in which others undertake effective caring interventions, such as our professional colleagues or informal carers.

Noticing the effects of cues and interactions on ourselves

We have learned that some interactions trigger within us certain responses. In Chapter 4 for example we found that identification with particular patients and objects can act as triggers and affect our emotional balance. We may be reminded of someone close to us or of some other aspect of our own life. Noticing and articulating these feelings may help us to care for ourselves and avoid compassion fatigue or distancing ourselves and becoming 'hard'. In doing so, we will be better able to remain caring in our approach to others.

We also found that with some patients we may establish an immediate rapport, in other words we 'click'. This may be beneficial in that it helps us to interact with a degree of ease but it can be problematic if we fail to notice that we may be moving outside parameters of our professional relationship.

We also need to notice how we are reacting to situations or to others and learn from both our positive and negative emotions. There are examples throughout the book of students and nurses who have learned a great deal from their negative but common emotions of guilt, dislike, anger and perhaps even disgust. We must recognise that we all have irrational and unrealistic thoughts at times and accept that we have a 'shadow side'. Nurses are not miracle workers or angels and the stories have helped us to understand that we need to learn to be able to cope with disappointment or any other negative feelings we might have. We have found that we should also recognise that what we think we might be like in the future (our 'possible selves') can be not only motivational but also based on hidden and sometimes irrational fears.

Noticing is an integral part of self-awareness, essential if we are to make rational judgements of our capabilities and reactions. We have suggested that we need to apply the same kind of critical analysis to ourselves as that which we use in our academic work. Indeed, the 'art of noticing' has been described by Boud and Walker (1990) as a principal component of reflection.

Noticing indicators of burnout and recognising the effects stress can have on patient care

Nurses experience all kinds of demanding situations and pressures which can lead to excessive stress. We have highlighted the importance of recognising and managing this and of looking after ourselves by developing the ability to 'bounce back' when meeting challenges or adversity (see Chapter 7). You will also notice the effects of particularly stressful periods on colleagues and we need to pay attention to emotional and behavioural cues which may indicate this. It is particularly important to notice when care is adversely affected because of this and seek help so appropriate action can be taken. As a member of a multi-professional team, noticing indicators of stress is an important way of caring for each other.

Caring by doing

This is the aspect that demonstrates to others our skills in caring. All aspects of the framework are interrelated (or are bonded) to each other and help reveal what caring is really all about. We must undertake various tasks and activities with a high level of practical expertise and skill, but without the 'artistry' required for holistic care for the person, which has been illuminated by the caring indicators, our nursing actions may fall short of what service users need and expect. Caring relationships are founded on good, safe practice. This means engaging in life-long learning and ongoing professional development to ensure we provide effective, skilful and safe care. We can only do this, however, if we care for ourselves effectively.

Preparing the ground for, and maintaining, caring relationships

Trust is an essential requirement for a caring relationship. As we have seen from the stories, in nursing this may have to be established within a very short period of time. This does not necessarily mean that the relationship between nurse and patient has to be at a very deep level, although as we have learned on many occasions interactions can become very meaningful. This is in line with Bassett (2002) who concludes that special 'bonds' may or may not occur between nurse and patient and that although closeness brings with it mutual benefits without this 'good' nursing care can still be given. However, we have found evidence that caring behaviours are important from the very start of interactions with patients and their relatives (whether they become 'deep' or remain at a 'superficial' level). Our indicators confirmed there are benefits to be gained from participating in informal social exchange and in simple acts of kindness which show others we are interested in and value them. We can develop trust and provide reassurance by being available and giving other people confidence both in our technical skills and in our ability to listen to and help them. We have seen the importance of responding to the concerns and distress of patients and their families and helping to reduce their pain, whether it is physical, emotional or spiritual.

Indicators also highlight the importance of interventions which help each service user to develop and retain a sense of personal worth, and feelings of acceptability and hope. We must promote and maintain caring relationships by engaging in anti-discriminatory practice and in doing so help others to maintain their self-respect and dignity. We have found that caring can be a spiritual union in which deep experience is shared and that we can help others in their search for comfort, meaning and hope. Respecting their religious beliefs, facilitating the meeting of their needs and practices is part of the caring process.

Much can be achieved through engaging in skilled verbal and non-verbal communication, responding and attending to detail in a 'care-ful' way. It is of particular importance to listen to how people describe their situation and lived experience. In this way we 'tune in' to them and use and develop our skills of empathy. The stories give us a great deal of information about how nurses can turn their compassion into effective nursing actions, for example the ways in which they help to change distressing situations into more manageable ones. This may include helping others to adapt and cope with change and to function at their optimal level.

Understanding and supporting informal carers

The importance of entering into equitable and non-patronising partnerships with informal carers has been highlighted in many of the stories. In order for effective multi-professional, multi-agency care to succeed, patients and carers need to be of central importance. There are often competing demands on carers and we found that professionals must engage in activities which take into account the whole 'family' and provide emotional support for them as required, particularly if they have to adapt and cope with change. Working in partnership with informal carers means valuing and using their knowledge and skills. It could also involve teaching and supporting them so that they can achieve quite complex practical skills and helping them to know how to access and negotiate for other resources. In this way people who are providing significant care can be helped to gain and share knowledge and 'power'. They are then more likely to retain the benefits of caring and continue to provide this essential part of the care continuum.

Engaging in critical analysis of practice

Throughout the previous chapters, we have made the point that a caring nurse engages in critical and analytical reflection. In this way they can gain knowledge for and from practice. Reflection on stories has demonstrated how much we can learn from seemingly small every-day occurrences as well as life-threatening and disturbing events. It is through examination and analysis that we find new ways of 'seeing' and 'doing', vital for compassionate and effective practice. It also helps us uncover aspects of caring which might otherwise be hidden, for example as we saw in Charlie and Bella's story in Chapter 4, effective communication was achieved by engaging in a 'dance of rhythmic harmony'. Critical analysis of this practice situation using academic perspectives helped with our understanding. Reflecting on and sharing stories such as this, help us to uncover and pass on tacit or hidden practice knowledge, articulating and adding to our caring skills. Critical reflection also helps us to uncover our capabilities and areas for further development. Throughout the book we have described various techniques and strategies we can use for this including using peer support, group discussion, reflective journals and the use of imagery and metaphor.

Caring for yourself and influencing the working environment

We have noted that in order to care for others we have to be nurtured ourselves. As we have seen, individual reflection with the help of a 'critical' friend or colleagues will help us to gain self-understanding and the confidence to overcome our fears, misconceptions and misgivings. The support we gain from our peers, family and friends should not be underestimated so we need to make time for them and for wider pursuits which help us to maintain equilibrium through achieving a healthy work-life balance. If we neglect these important aspects of our lives we will not be able to care effectively or influence a working environment which is conducive to care.

Over one hundred years ago, Florence Nightingale considered that the most important aspect of nursing was to create the conditions under which a person could be healed by nature or by God (Nightingale, 1969). An environment can be healing if we care 'with' as well as care 'for' a patient and their family. Then we are, as Barker and Buchanan-Barker (2004) suggest, helping individuals to grow and develop by giving them literal and metaphorical 'nourishment' which lies at the root of nursing. To do this we need to draw on both the scientific and the artistic knowledge base for nursing. Service users need to feel safe and are entitled to skilled, evidence-based interventions. A caring nurse therefore needs to keep up to date, be highly skilled in technical procedures and be able to understand, utilise and evaluate the relevance of research findings. The caring indicators have particularly highlighted the importance of the art of nursing, since that is the aspect of caring which is so easily taken for granted or not understood. As we have seen however, this is not an indulgence but an imperative and should have equal weight with the science of nursing. Expertise in technical skills without attending to the person can be detrimental to the healing process just as would 'sympathy' without a knowledgeable skills base.

The practice setting can influence the way we care for and with others. If the atmosphere is one of distrust, disorganisation and lacks warmth and collegiality, it will be stressful for both the cared-for as well as those providing the care. Even as a student nurse you can make a contribution to this influential environment - not only by the way in which you contribute to care but also by the ways in which you support and work with colleagues, keep 'cool' in stressful situations, use humour appropriately and assist in developing others as well as yourself.

Summary

In this chapter we have provided an overview of the caring indicators summarised at the end of each chapter. These were derived from stories told to us by patients and their relatives, students and qualified nurses. We found there were numerous indicators which often confirmed research findings and perspectives from academic literature but were brought to life and reassessed for their relevance to caring in practice. We found that categorising them into four main themes helped to clarify and encapsulate what a caring nurse is and does. These were:

1. Being and becoming
2. Overcoming obstacles
3. Noticing
4. Doing.

The initial BOND framework for caring could be used to develop your understanding further. Remember that frameworks are there just to help us; they are not complete answers but can be useful tools for developing our understanding and behaviour. Although the aspects of caring we have outlined are applicable to many situations and contexts in which nurses presently work, the world of practice continues to change dramatically. Our caring skills need to evolve to meet the challenge of these changes and that is why it is so important to ensure your analytical and reflective caring discourse continues.

Looking forward

In Chapter 9, we will review the journey of learning we have made throughout this book and consider the importance of continuing to maintain caring as a key aspect of nursing, whatever the future holds for the profession.

Activity

Look for caring moments in practice and consider one of these, for example an interaction between a qualified nurse and a patient or carer. Try using the BOND framework to help with your reflections and draw on relevant literature which will help you achieve a deeper analysis.

References

Abraham, R (2004) Emotional competence as antecedent to performance: a contingency framework. *Genetic, Social and General Psychology Monographs* **130**, 117-143.

Barker, P and Buchanan-Barker, P (2004) Caring as a craft. *Nursing Standard* **19**, 17-18.

Bassett, C (2002) Nurses' perceptions of care and caring. *International Journal of Nursing Practice* **8**, 8-15.

Boud, D and Walker, D (1990) Making the most of experience. *Studies in Continuing Education* **12**, 61-80.

Jacelon, C (1997) The trait and process of resilience. *Journal of Advanced Nursing* **25**, 123-129.

Jackson, D, Firtko, A and Edenborough, M (2007) Personal resilience as a strategy for surviving and thriving in the face of workplace adversity: a literature review. *Journal of Advanced Nursing* **60**, 1-9.

McQueen, A (2004) Emotional intelligence in nursing work. *Journal of Advanced Nursing* **47**, 101-108.

Nightingale, F (1969) *Notes on Nursing: what it is and what it is not.* New York: Dover. (First published in 1860.)

Tusaie, K and Dyer, J (2004) Resilience: a historical review of the construct. *Holistic Nursing Practice* **18**, 3-8.

Chapter 9

Looking back and moving forward

LEARNING OBJECTIVES

The purpose by the end of this chapter is to have an understanding of:

1. The contribution stories can make in uncovering the many dimensions of caring.
2. The importance of ensuring that the value of caring knowledge and practice is not lost within organisational changes and shifting professional bodies.
3. The value of extending the caring capacity within the working environment.

Introduction

In this final chapter we will review our journey and consider again what we can learn about the nature of caring if we use stories from patients, carers and nurses for reflective analysis. However, we will also remind ourselves about the hazards and pitfalls of storytelling.

Learning about caring must be an ongoing process and therefore we need to see this within the context of changes in the way in which care is provided and delivered over the coming years. We know that qualified nurses are increasingly expected to develop effective leadership, management and entrepreneurial skills and we will consider the place for emotional work within a business context.

Reviewing our journey

In this book, we have journeyed together and begun to unravel some of the many dimensions of caring which we see as encompassing both the art and the science of nursing. Writing this book has reinforced for us, that the artistry of nursing is highly important and must be integrated into the application of scientific knowledge and technological skills. This is the only way we can provide holistic care. Scientific knowledge or the ability to engage in complex technological skills is exciting and has high status but the art of caring may be taken for granted, not well articulated and its significance overlooked. We hope you have found that, in the same way as they have for us, the stories have led you to appreciate that sometimes even everyday, basic tasks create important opportunities for caring, which can be equally as engaging and therapeutic as undertaking complex technological interventions.

The stories have been central in uncovering the art of nursing. Tschudin (1999: 198) defines an artist as not only one who paints, sculpts or is a creative cook but anyone who undertakes 'any gesture or act that takes us beyond ourselves and opens our physical and inner eyes to something more than the obvious'. The stories from service users, carers, student and qualified nursing staff have done just this - enabling us to see things in a new light and have generated new understandings of things which might otherwise have been hidden from view. You may have been surprised at the number of caring indicators that emerged at the end of each chapter as a result of critically analysing our stories. These led us to create the BOND framework outlined in Chapter 8. You will remember that we categorised the caring indicators into four main themes to help to clarify and encapsulate what a caring nurse is and does. These were:

1. Being and becoming
2. Overcoming obstacles
3. Noticing
4. Doing.

Our thoughts about the importance of stories

To think about

Think again about how stories have always been part of your life and how they contribute to your professional working life and development. Make a few notes and compare your considerations with ours.

Compare your considerations with ours

Like us you may have thought about how important stories were to you as a child. We expect you can remember many of the favourite stories of your childhood. Some of them, like fables, had a very strong moral message. Stories also came in different forms such as in nursery rhymes and poems. Songs also contain stories and some of these may evoke strong memories or emotional attachments. You will have recognised that stories are all around us and an integral part of our everyday lives – perhaps when we are telling others about the good times we have had or a particularly memorable event. The media abounds with stories, some 'true' and some completely fabricated. This may all seem very obvious but we wanted to underline the significance of their influence on our everyday experience, perceptions, attitudes, values and behaviour. In other words they are part of our culture and help form social constructs about important issues such as our views of what is right and what is wrong; how we may view (construct) old age, immigration, people with learning disabilities and mental health problems, and perhaps risks to children and of body image.

As in everyday life, stories have an important influence on the way in which we perceive and therefore construct nursing. From the very beginning of the book, we learned about the value of stories as rich learning experiences in our professional life and through them we began our journey into a discourse about caring. From the stories we were able to identify significant caring moments which occurred in busy traumatic periods but also in everyday situations. For example in Chapter 1, we saw the contribution students could make in the caring process such as in the story of Jo who, as a first year student, was able to send out a powerful message that she cared by using her natural warm, informal communication skills. By using stories as a focus for our reflection we learned that we can critically explore our practice including our myths, beliefs and values and increase our knowledge of caring. We also saw the value of using stories from those being 'cared for' in order to be more knowledgeable about their perceptions of the caring process and be in a better position to learn from and transform nursing care. Stories also helped us to see the importance of helping informal carers to maintain rewarding relationships with those for whom they care so they are not overwhelmed by the demands of providing care.

Stories helped us to look again at partnerships in nursing care and we saw that these can be very rewarding for both nurse and patient – a process of giving and receiving – and through deeper analysis we were able to uncover the significance of being aware of and accepting emotional gifts from others. We came to the conclusion that if we want to achieve true partnerships with patients, we have to acknowledge and value their contribution to our own personal and professional growth. For example Ellie's story and reflections about her interactions with George (Chapter 2) helped us to gain more understanding of what it really means to care and to see caring as a two-way process.

In Chapter 3, we looked at both caring and uncaring moments in practice. The stories we identified of uncaring or negative attitudes may not have led to official complaints or investigations into professional misconduct but unfortunately occur almost everyday in practice and are mainly the result of unthinking or uninformed care rather than deliberate cruelty. In some cases these incidents caused extreme distress and may have resulted in long-term effects on service users and their families. To overcome such difficulties, we concluded that nurses need to focus on developing a heightened awareness by listening to and 'hearing' patients' lived experiences, including acknowledging the contribution of the expert patient. In this chapter, the patients emphasised how much they valued 'simple' acts of kindness, which all health care staff may easily overlook.

The relevance of acknowledging and using our emotions as a resource for developing our caring skills was discussed, and throughout the book we have seen how stories can act as an important starting point for reflection. We found that the world of nursing can be demanding but may also be intensely satisfying. We saw how nurses helped patients to overcome problems related to self-image with the story of Charlie and Bella illustrating this (Chapter 4). Charlie's story helped us learn more about the part assumptions and emotions can play in the way in which we as nurses make judgements and behave. In other stories there were examples of how identification with particular patients and objects can act as triggers and affect our emotional balance. We saw the importance of using opportunities for reflective learning which could help us gain more understanding of the parameters of our professional relationship with service users and their families.

In Chapter 5, we found that holistic care is not easy within changing political, economic and social contexts but can be helped if we work closely with relatives and their families in identifying not only problems but also family strengths and resources. Recognition that, as professionals, we are often only one small part of a continuum of care will make us more alert to the importance of ensuring that we work with informal carers. Paying attention to what people say about their lived experiences of illness or disability, of providing care and being cared for, will help us to bring into effect the most important aspect, that of truly caring partnerships.

In the latter part of the book we used stories which enabled us to focus more closely on how we can learn from our emotions. For example in Chapter 6 we used several stories from practice to discuss how reflection can increase our self-awareness and considered the ways in which we might be more analytical about ourselves. We showed how we could use metaphors and images to help us understand ourselves and others more. We also explored the notion of emotional intelligence and its place in our professional development including competencies such as self-awareness, motivation, self-regulation, empathy and skilfulness in relationships. We stressed the importance of finding ways of developing these aspects if we are to maintain and enhance, and even transform, caring.

We went on to discuss some of demanding situations and pressures which can lead to excessive stress (Chapter 7). We highlighted the importance of recognising and managing this and of looking after ourselves as professional carers. If you have the ability to 'bounce back' when meeting challenges or adversity, you will be less likely to be at risk of becoming overwhelmed and to experience emotional exhaustion. This emotional resilience will develop if you are able to see solutions as well as problems or difficulties and acknowledge and use the strengths and resources you have within yourself and within others. We saw how Joanne used a solution-focused approach to help Lara. We suggested that this could also be useful in the development of others including patients/clients and their families. At times our strengths and resources may be ignored or undervalued, such as the ways in which we use our creativity and the impact of the close and 'spiritual' relationships we develop with patients and clients. These all help us to improve and sustain our 'artistry' in caring and to value it as the central aspect of nursing.

To think about

Stories are very powerful and very useful but there are some hazards and pitfalls associated with them.

✦ What do you think they are? Make particular reference to your professional life and make a few notes. If you get stuck you may find Chapter 1 helpful.

Compare your considerations with ours

We hope you will find similarities but don't worry if you have come to some different conclusions. Stories are told for a purpose. The way we tell and reflect on our stories depends on who is listening to us. An easy way of considering this is to use the key words of what, when, why, where, how and who. As we noted in Chapter 1, stories are socially reconstructed and reflect the content and the expected audience (Mishler, 1991). The stories you use for your reflections as part of your educational course or in clinical supervision are likely to take on a different form from 'storytelling' occurring with a colleague in an informal setting. We think that although using your stories to describe your practice experience is useful as part of an academic exercise – in that you can learn valuable lessons from integrating theory and practice and thinking again about your performance – there is a pitfall in that you may be constrained by academic marking criteria and so feel unable to disclose or address particular strong emotional feelings that you have. You may therefore submit a 'sanitised' account. Many of our students overcame this by finding that they gained most help from sharing their powerful personal stories with their peers or a trusted colleague.

The power of stories can be a disadvantage as well as an advantage. Horror stories or biased views about people and situations can engender fear and distrust. They may form the basis of professional gossip and of unfortunate categorisations such as the 'unpopular' patient, relative, nurse or colleague. Perceptions of particular student placements may be based on one particular scary story or a myth. However, as we have seen in this book, it is helpful to become sensitive and to be honest about what might be our tendency to exaggerate or emphasise (to make the story more interesting or to get sympathy). We will then be able to uncover prejudices or biases which might affect our relationships and behaviour.

We can also get stuck within the emotional content of stories and therefore not use them as effectively as we might if we do not reflect on them at a deeper analytical level. To do this we need to look for a wide variety of perspectives and different forms of evidence. We (as authors) recognised this when we began to consider writing this book about caring in nursing. We knew that any attempt at a simple definition would be inadequate and that the stories would evoke a variety of emotions associated with caring (and indeed uncaring) behaviour. These could be more effectively examined through the use of a wide variety of resources and our examination included theoretical perspectives. We hope that, like us, you have found how interesting this can be.

Stepping into the future

To think about

+ Identify and list changes which you think are likely to occur over the next few years and which could have an impact on the way in which nursing care is provided.
+ Pause for a moment to think and then compare your thoughts with the discussion which follows.

It is difficult to predict as the world changes continuously: economically, politically, socially and environmentally. However, our list includes the likelihood of a number of issues.

Demographic changes – the population in the UK is likely to continue changing as the number of people over the age of 60 increases. There is also likely to be greater movement of individuals across countries particularly within the European Union. An ageing nursing workforce along with competition for experienced nurses to be employed in other countries such as the USA, Canada and Australia will have an impact on the UK's nursing workforce.

There will be increases in the number of people with complex health and social needs which will include those with learning disabilities and young adults and children. Other increases such as the number of people with different forms of dementia will affect most areas of nursing. In all these areas funding issues for health and social care will continue and there will remain a focus on value for money and proven effectiveness.

There will be continued emphasis on primary and community health particularly related to preventative interventions to promote health, for example in reducing the number of people who are obese. People will be expected to take a greater role in their own health management so may need help to be able to access and evaluate health information, e.g. from the internet.

There will more expectation that people with chronic/long-term conditions will be supported so they are able to 'self-care'. In addition, there is likely to be more emphasis on pathways of care which will cut across primary and secondary care. Increasing attention will be given to patient experience and how care is managed. There will be more care provided closer to home and within the home environment.

Increases in technology and scientific and medical knowledge will result in ongoing pressures for more specialisation for all health care workers but particularly for nurses. At the same time, there will be consumer pressure for quality care, and recognition of human rights will continue. There will be a drive for more collaborative approaches including more involvement of patients and carers and an increase in patient choice.

We looked for further ideas from a discussion paper commissioned by the Nursing and Midwifery Council undertaken by Longley *et al.* (2007) who considered a number of options for change in pre-registration education of nursing to meet the challenges of the changes such as those mentioned above by 2015. They suggested that nurses will need to be more flexible and that there would be an increase in the number undertaking specialised and advanced roles. Because care will be focused in the community they stressed the importance of working within and across patient pathways and of effective multidisciplinary teamworking. They also proposed that these changes should be reflected in nursing career pathways. They outlined the possibility of several key opportunities for nurses, including directing and leading care, both within and outside the NHS, using entrepreneurial skills and that nurses could be at the forefront of initiatives in public health and preventative medicine. To do all this they suggest that 'Nurses will be required to have a high level of knowledge, critical thinking, and autonomy at registration' (Longley *et al.*, 2007: 34). Debates about future roles and responsibilities will continue and we need to engage with them if nurses are to influence the future of nursing.

Our work has shown us that service users expect that nurses and others who provide care are caring individuals and this is a key reason why we all came into nursing. In the future, we must ensure that we do not lose our caring knowledge and skills with any expansion of nursing roles so that we are able to keep caring as a central component. We must therefore continue to articulate caring behaviours and demonstrate what difference caring makes to a variety of outcomes including meeting government and organisational targets and in evaluating quality of care and the experiences of service users. In the future it would seem that more direct care may be provided by health care assistants (or their equivalent). An important part of your leadership role in the future (and one we believe must not be forgotten within a business-orientated, evidence-based health care system with its myriad pressures and preoccupations) will be to share with them knowledge and skills you have about the art of caring. In this way caring will survive and grow.

Extending our caring capacity – recognising the importance of emotional capital

To think about

Qualified nurses are increasingly expected to develop effective leadership, management and entrepreneurial skills.

✦ Do you think there is a place for emotional work within a business orientation?
✦ Pause for a moment to think and then compare your thoughts with the discussion which follows.

As we have seen from each chapter in this book, the emotional work of nurses is an important asset which can be taken for granted or overlooked. It is difficult to measure, but the term 'capital' is used in economics and management to define the assets, resources and relative wealth of a particular group or commodity. It is heart-warming that there is increasing recognition of the importance of the value of what is described as emotional capital in business management. Gendron (2004), an economist and expert in human resources, considers that this involves emotional competencies within individuals which are necessary for personal, professional and also for organisational development. She also suggests that these competencies are vital for social and economic success and therefore asserts that emotional capital must be taken into account seriously by policy-makers, practitioners and business organisations. She explains it this way:

> 'Emotional capital is the set (resource) of emotional competencies which gives individuals and organizations the ability to use emotions to help individuals at solving problems and living a more effective life and the organisation at facing economic and social changes and being successful and surviving in the new economics world. ... It is the head working with the heart and the hands. ... For a full and ethical use of Human Resource with a big H, that implies taking into account the three Hs of each individual: Hands, Head and Heart.' (Gendron, 2004: 31)

What she is saying is important for us in that the emotional capital of the caring nurse is an important resource which needs to recognised, nurtured and developed. The notion of emotional capital as an important resource in the 'hard-nosed' business world reinforces the importance of perceiving caring as an asset. In nursing, this may be taken for granted and may not always be recognised unless it is missing. As a student you should be proud of giving emotional support to others (service users, relatives or colleagues) just as you are pleased about being able to use highly technical skills. We consider that this emotional work is as demanding and as influential. If you continue to value the emotional work which you do – for yourself and others – once you are qualified you will use strategies which encourage and nurture this within your team. By doing so you will enhance your working environment and create a caring culture.

Summary

The nature of nursing work gives us a valid reason to interact with patients and their families. Caring is not unique to nursing but our presence with people during periods of their lives when they are feeling most vulnerable provides unique opportunities such as when we recognise and respond to distress, pain, misunderstandings, loss of hope or meaning. We need to retain the benefits of our traditional 'hands-on' approaches, particularly if we move away from providing fundamental care but are undertaking more highly specialised and complex interventions. These changes will provide us with new opportunities which we can use to continue to draw on both the art and the science of nursing to express our caring skills.

This will be an important challenge for nurses in the future, just as it is for us today, as we struggle to retain caring relationships within organisations which are increasingly outcome-driven and have considerable economic constraints upon them. We have to develop our skills in providing and presenting a wide range of evidence concerning the difference which our caring skills make to the experiences of service users and also to the outcomes of their care. These will be important aspects for you as you take on roles in leadership, management and research and develop skills required for quality assurance and evidence-based practice.

Nursing has an exciting future as it responds to the changing nature of health and social care to meet changing demographic trends and service user needs and expectations. There will an increasing crossing-over of traditional professional boundaries and a blurring between health and social care. As nurses we need to respond effectively and creatively to these changes but also we must have the determination to keep caring at the very heart of nursing whatever the future brings.

Activity

Think of ways in which you will endeavour to keep caring at the heart of your practice. This may mean looking back (such as by using a reflective journal), but also looking forward. For example, think of ways in which care can be planned to truly reflect effective partnerships with patients and their carers. This could be whether you are working within your own discipline or with multi-profesional or muti-agency colleagues.

References

Gendron, B (2004) **Why emotional capital matters in education and in labour? Toward an optimal exploitation of human capital and knowledge management.** *Les Cahiers de la Maison des Sciences Economiques, série rouge, n° 113*. Université Panthéon-Sorbonne, Paris, pp. 37 **Accessible on:** www.en.wilkipedia.org/wiki/Emotional-capital (last accessed 29 March 2008).

Longley, M, Shaw, C and Dolan, G (2007) *Nursing: Towards 2015. Alternative scenarios for healthcare, nursing and nurse education in the UK in 2015*. Welsh Institute for Health and Social Care, University of Glamorgan.

Mishler, E (1991) "Once upon a time...". *Journal of Narrative and Life History* **2**, 3, 101-108.

Tschudin, V (1999) *Nurses Matter: Reclaiming our professional identity*. Basingstoke: Macmillan.

Index

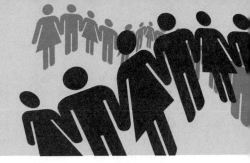